Stop Using Your Mind

GET HEALTHIER AND HAPPIER IN SEVEN DAYS USING MEDITATION AND DIET

Stop Using Your Mind

GET HEALTHIER AND HAPPIER IN SEVEN DAYS USING MEDITATION AND DIET

Celia Ko

AWARD WINNING AUTHOR

Copyright © 2025 by Celia Ko

All rights reserved. No part of this publication may be reproduced, distributed, or transmitted in any form or by any means, including, photocopying,recording, or other electronic or mechanical methods, without the prior written permission of the copyright owner and the publisher, except in the case of brief quotations embodied in critical reviews and certain other noncommercial uses permitted by copyright law. For permission requests, write to the publisher, addressed "Attention: Permissions Coordinator," at the address below.

CITIOFBOOKS, INC.
3736 Eubank NE Suite A1
Albuquerque, NM 87111-3579
www.citiofbooks.com
Hotline: 1 (877) 389-2759
Fax: 1 (505) 930-7244

Ordering Information:
Quantity sales. Special discounts are available on quantity purchases by corporations, associations, and others. For details, contact the publisher at the address above.

Printed in the United States of America.
ISBN-13: Paperback 979-8-89391-773-4
eBook 979-8-89391-774-1

Library of Congress Control Number: 2025913045

Table of Contents

Acknowledgements i
Foreword iii

Chapter 1: Why Meditation? 1
Chapter 2: The Way of Meditation 13
Chapter 3: Healthy Mind, Healthy Body 26
Chapter 4: The Importance of Sleep 38
Chapter 5: The Color of Food 48
Chapter 6: Four Seasons of Health 59
Chapter 7: The Difference Between Sleep and Meditation 71
Chapter 8: Healthier and Happier Every Day 82

*Thank you, dear reader, for being here.
I hope you now are able to use these valuable tools
to help you live happier and healthier each and every day.*

Acknowledgements

For Master Shi Wanxing, whose wisdom gives me guidance in life. For my family and dear friends, whose love and support will never cease to warm my heart.

FOREWORD

Do you ever wonder what life would be like if you woke up every morning excited for the day? Do you feel like you are missing something? You look around you and see happy people who appear to have it all. Maybe you once thought that wasn't possible for you, but now you are beginning to wake up. There is a part of you that knows you deserve all that this universe has to offer. Living a happy, healthy and fulfilling life is in fact within your grasp, and you are done waiting for permission to get out there and grab it.

Are you ready to take your life back? Are you ready to take control? Are you ready to do the work? If you answered yes to all of the above, then you have come to the right book. Celia Ko generously shares her simple formula for living a happy and healthy life. She brings together her knowledge of Chinese medicine, meditation, and yoga into one simple practice that is easy to understand and practice.

Celia has spent many years helping people stop using their minds in meditation, ultimately raising their energy through the reduction of anxiety and stress. No matter how reluctant you might be, she has tools to help you develop a daily meditation practice that not only improves mood and focus but also helps aid in sleeping restfully through the night. You are guaranteed to find inspiration within the chapters of Stop Using Your Mind, that will see you through any resistance you might face when meeting the challenges of changing your habits head on.

One of the greatest aspects of Celia's writing is how easy it is to read.

She takes complex concepts and breaks them down into understandable and actionable steps. From easy to follow meditation exercises to delicious recipes, she helps you achieve success in developing more healthy habits. In her writing she also shares some personal stories, including challenges faced and how they were overcome, from her practices. Through these stories, she creates a shared experience to help you see how you too can achieve your goals.

Get ready to embark on your own amazing journey. You are here. You are ready. With Stop Using Your Mind and Celia Ko's incredible teachings, you have everything you need right now to live happy and healthy every single day of your life going forward. Today is the day to step onto the path of pure joy. I promise you; you will not regret picking up this book!

Raymond Aaron
New York Times Bestselling Author

Chapter 1

Why Meditation?

"Feelings come and go like clouds in a windy sky. Conscious breathing is my anchor."

– Thich Nhat Hanh

Meditation will transform your life if you allow yourself to stop using your mind. It is that simple. Calming your thoughts and focusing on your breath will bring a sense of calm and peace to your days. We live on this Earth, but we spend 100% of that time in our own heads. Everything you see, feel, touch, taste, and experience is done so through the lens of your thoughts. If those thoughts are consistently filled with worry, anger, and anxiety, this is how you experience our world. How can you truly expect to experience the happy moments authentically when your thoughts are getting in the way?

Take a moment and think back to a time when you wanted to feel good about what was happening in your life. Maybe you were on vacation at a beautiful resort, or your family was throwing you a party to celebrate your birthday. Looking around you, you knew you should feel good. You knew you should be happy. But your thoughts were pulling you out of the moment. Maybe you were worried about an issue at work. Maybe you were upset with your partner for some small task they forgot to complete. Maybe you were thinking about how life just wasn't what you thought it would be. Do you see what I mean with this example?

Your thoughts have the ability to take away your happiness. Your thoughts can change your perspective. Your thoughts can cloud your judgement. Basically, your thoughts have power. Sometimes it may feel like you are drowning in your daily life. There is so much work to be done. There is so much to worry about. You might be reading this and thinking that meditation won't help because the problems in your life are real and your thoughts can't change that.

I agree with you in one regard, that often the problems you face are real. However, you can change how you react to them by changing the way you think about them. Regardless of what is happening in the world around you, you can achieve peace in your life.

In this book, I will share with you the benefits of meditation for both your physical and mental health. In this busy world where you are asked to achieve so much in so little time, you can often feel stressed, anxious, and burnt out. Learning to simply just be with your breath will help you not only gain perspective on what is important to you; it will help you find gratitude for yourself, your family, and all of the abundance you have in your life. I will then connect this concept to the importance of nutrition and sleep to help you achieve happiness in your daily life.

In recent years, meditation has come to see some popularity, which can be good, but it can also be bad. There is a lot of misinformation out there. A lot of it is pertaining to even the simplest of details, like how to sit, the environment you meditate in, and even how to breathe properly. I will share with you the simple and effective techniques to help you learn how to meditate with ease.

A common misconception is that it is difficult to turn off the mind. This is not true. Many people think that they just can't do it, when they really haven't tried. Meditation can be easy, but it does take discipline. Once you achieve the ability to sit quietly with yourself in the moment, you will learn peace. Peace in your thoughts. Peace in your perspective. Peace in your feelings. This sense of peace will allow you to find a calm approach to daily life.

Who Am I?

I was born in 1966 in China. At the age of seven, I was appointed by the Chinese government to be a gymnast. In America, parents often put their children in things like gymnastics or dance or sports to give them the opportunity to learn what they want to do with their lives, or many these activities are meant to be fun and social.

This was not what gymnastics was for me. I was meant to win. I was being trained to be one of the best gymnasts in the world from a very young age. I think this is one of the first times in my life I remember experiencing true hardship. Children who are appointed to be trained as gymnasts are isolated and forced to move to a specialized school. The training is grueling, both physically and mentally.

After a few years of this training, my family was able to move to Hong Kong. China had opened the doors for people to be able to travel back to their hometowns. I was born into a very wealthy family. My father was born in Indonesia but was sent to China to go and live with grandparents. He had lived in China ever since.

Moving to Hong Kong introduced the Western world to me. Without knowing a single letter in the English alphabet, I attended an English learning school in addition to the regular elementary school. I managed to finish 6 years of English lessons within 2 years.

The Hong Kong educational system at that time required elementary students to take public (open) examinations on all subjects that were given to all students. Then the students had to fill out a form to pick the school they wanted. The department of education would put all the grades a student got into a computer system and let the computer generate a result. If the student got good grades for all subjects, the student would be granted entrance to their first choice. Otherwise, the student had to take the risk of being assigned randomly by the computer system to the worst school, because if your grades were not good enough to enter into the best school, the computer would not assign you to go to the second ranking school. Therefore, the student had to make sure what his/her level was and what school would best fit them. I was secretly told by my English teacher that I should pick the best English girls' school in Hong Kong because my overall grades were the top three out of all the girls in the graduate classes.

I thrive on knowledge. In this life, I desire growth. Every day, I wake up at 5:00 a.m. and fill my time with meditation, work, and learning. I have never watched a moment of television in my life. I love to read. I love to travel. I love to catch up on my English. I love to learn. Most importantly, I love to be a light in a world that can often feel dark.

I first ran away from my father in my teenage years. I had already faced much hardship in my young life, and I was searching for peace. It has always been my goal to live a peaceful life. At the age of seventeen, I flew to Taiwan by myself, only to be called back home to the family after my father had a heart attack. Even though I was most certainly not his favored child, I was the only one who could run his business for him. During this time, I also had to finish my final years of school. After form 6, my father kicked me out of the house again. He had a new girlfriend and twin boys to occupy his time.

I flew back to Taiwan for college. Yet, I always wanted to go to the USA to get a higher education. I was done with Taiwan and needed to find my way in the world. I had a bigger dream while my father and my grandparents wanted me to get married to a rich guy so that they would no longer be responsible for me. They emphasized to me that giving money to a girl to have a higher education was just like pouring a bucket of water on the ground. You could never get the water back from the ground, and they were not stupid! They added that because they were smart businesspeople, they would not invest money in a dead product, which was a girl. After she got married, she would not carry their family name, and their own wealthy family had no position for a girl with another family name after she got married.

A friend of mine had moved to Hawaii and invited me to join her. Without my father's blessing, I decided to take her up on her offer, and I never left Hawaii after that. I became an international student in Hawaii. I met my husband. Together, we have run a successful business of our own for the past 32 years. We have a son who is now 30, and we are both so proud of his accomplishments in the film industry. I believe he has done so well because of the way we supported him.

All of this said, life in Hawaii has not been without its hardships.

As hard as I tried, my mother-in-law never liked me. For much of my life, I have sought peace, and this caused me great sadness. Reflecting back on the time I spent living in those moments, I know that its greatest lesson was that in order to have peace in my life, I needed to find peace within myself. Life gives you the experiences you need, to become the person you need to be to live your purpose. Everything is working for you, even though it doesn't feel like it a lot of the time.

In my life, I have understood suffering. I have experienced hardship from a young age. The most important lesson meditation has taught me is that I have the ability to turn my suffering into power. It is my strength. For the longest time, I had never understood what the point of my suffering was. From my young years in China at the gymnastics school, to the first time I ran away from home in my teens, to making my own way in America with very little money, I didn't understand why I was meant to struggle so much. But now I do. I understand that all I have been through has led me to this moment. I am powerful. I know my strength. I am happy. I have learned how to overcome my worry, my sadness, and my anger, and how to breathe. It is through breath that I make my way back to myself, to my strength.

My life purpose is to guide 10 million people in discovering the way to a happy life. Through all of the hardship, I have learned how to live in peace, both with myself and the world around me. I want the same for you. I know if you are able to achieve this, you will want to share it with others too. Together, we create a movement. Together, we make this world a better place for ourselves, our families, and our communities. Together, we too can make this world a more peaceful place. When you make decisions from a place of calm contentment, even in moments of turmoil, you can show others how to do the same. This is my purpose, and I am so glad you are here to join me on this journey.

Who Is My Inspiration?

The master who has inspired my meditation journey is Master Shi Wanxing. He is a monk and a teacher who isolated himself for seven years within the seclusion of a cave to meditate. This kind of dedication is inspiring, but this was his path. He did this so that he could share with the world what he learned.

I personally have no desire to spend seven years in a cave, so I am grateful for his teachings. His style combines the principles of Buddhism and Daoism. Life is not only a process of learning; it is also one of sharing love. Master Wanxing leads by example when it comes to sharing love. For him, it is about the unconditional love that he gives people. His core value in life is to make the world a better place.

Master Wanxing inspires people to be their own master. He has helped me and countless others around the world to end our own suffering by looking for the lessons in our hardships. Allowing yourself to see that everything you experience in life is a lesson, will help you find peace. When you find peace, you can help others to do the same. Only when you can become the sunshine, can you give warmth to others.

Everything that happens in life is the best thing to happen. Don't differentiate the bad and the good things that you came across. Accept all and appreciate all the setbacks and the difficulties that you have in life and treat them as great lessons. Send love to the ones who brought you hardship and thank them for being your great teachers in life.

Master Shi Wanxing has given me and so many others around the world the opportunity to experience the benefits of meditation. From him I learned to cultivate my own inner world through the use of breath. Once you know how to properly use your breath, you will change your life. His method of teaching meditation is simple and effective. I have used them myself for years now and I am excited to share them with you.

Many people in Western culture are wanting to try meditation because the word about its benefits have continued to spread. That said, there is now a lot of misinformation out there. With my work, I aim to spread the truth. I aim to help others understand what they need to know to develop an effective meditation practice.

I have been meditating for 5 years now. Every single day, I chant and meditate. I have combined this with healthy eating and getting a good night's sleep to achieve a happier and more peaceful existence.

What Will You Learn?

Ultimately, you will learn how to live a happier and more fulfilled life. My hope for everyone who chooses to read this book is that they find strength within themselves through breath. When you are able to stop using your mind, you give yourself an incredible gift: peace. You learn how to calm yourself. You learn how to release the stress, worry, regret, fear, and anxiety that is holding you in a place of sadness.

To begin your meditation practice, you will learn:

- The proper posture and why it is important.
- How to breathe.
- Why you should always make sure your environment is conducive to meditating properly.
- What chi is and why it is important.
- What clothing you should wear and why it is important.
- Why sleep is important.
- Why diet is important.
- The relationship of meditation, sleep, and diet for your happiness.

To begin getting a better night's sleep, you will learn:

- How to sleep with the cosmic energy of the sun and moon.
- How to set yourself up for a good night's sleep.
- What not to do before bed.
- How much sleep you need to feel rejuvenated in the morning.

To begin eating healthier, you will learn:
- How to improve your diet by applying seasonal food.
- How to use the five color rules for your diet.
- How to drink water properly on a daily basis.
- How to regulate the amount of food for your 3 meals in a day.
- The time that you should eat, according to the internal clock of your digestive system.
- How to fast if needed. Often, a fast is healthy practice after indulging over the holidays or a period of celebration.

The Benefits of Meditation, Sleeping Well, and a Healthy Diet

"The popularity of meditation is increasing as more people discover its benefits. Many people think of it as a way to reduce stress and develop concentration. People also use it to develop other beneficial habits and feelings, such as positive mood and outlook, self-discipline, healthy sleep patterns, and even increased pain tolerance."

– **Dr. Matthew Thorpe**

There are so many incredible benefits to meditation. I've already touched on one of the most important: to gain control of your thoughts and allow your mind some much needed rest. When your mind can rest, you can find peace. When you can find peace, you will make healthier choices for your body. Meditation brings you into the moment, allowing you to release your negative feelings about the past and your worries about the future. It reminds you to stay present in the reality of the moment.

In this moment, you are one human being walking through life. Your body is all connected. When your mind is at peace, your body feels healthy, and in the same way, when your body is healthy, your mind has an easier time finding peace.

So, what comes first? Meditating, healthier sleep patterns, or better nutrition? Neither! You can work on all of them at the same time. I believe, when you begin to work on one aspect of your life, you'll find that all of the connected parts of you feel this energy, and you will want to grow to live in a healthier place as well. I am going to begin our journey together by sharing my teachings on establishing an effective meditation practice, but you can also begin to think about your sleep patterns and diet at the same time.

Both your body and mind need rest to function at a high level. I have met many people who say they function well on as little as four hours of sleep a night, but I would argue that they are not functioning at their highest potential. I can't wait to share with you a very beneficial tool to help you achieve some of the best sleep you will have ever experienced in your life, which is understanding how to sleep with the cosmic energy of the sun and moon.

When you are exhausted and stressed, you might find yourself in a vicious cycle that you can't pull yourself out of. You don't feel good, so you make poor choices with your food. You eat late at night to fill an emotional void, and this stops you from having a good night's sleep. You wake up with low energy and in a low mood again the next day, causing you to once again make the same choices that you did the day before. The tools you will learn in the remainder of this chapter and the ones that follow will help you break that cycle.

Once you begin meditating, eating good food, and sleeping well, you will see how it's all connected. You will create a cycle of happiness for yourself that will be hard to break!

A Moment of Reflection

Before you get started on your practice, take some time to reflect on your goals and why they are important to you. Some people like to write out their responses in a journal; some type them up, and others just sit in quiet contemplation. The nice thing about writing out your responses is that you can revisit them when you are feeling like the work is too hard. Changing lifelong thought patterns and habits is challenging.

Think about it like a path in the grass. If many people walk the same path, it is easier. The grass doesn't grow as high. There are no bushes to push through or prickly vines to worry about. You don't have to think as much about it. You simply just walk the path you know, even if you may not want to walk this path any longer. There might be a beautiful tree whose shade you've wanted to enjoy for years, but every day you make the choice to walk the easy path. "Tomorrow," you say to yourself. "Tomorrow, I'll walk out into the thick field and make my way to that beautiful tree for a rest in the shade."

Your body and your brain will always find it easier to think the same things and choose the same actions it has been choosing for years, even though it doesn't feel good anymore. What it does feel is comfortable.

In the reflection exercise, you will be asked to get out of your comfort zone. Think big! Push yourself to understand what it is you truly want to achieve and how you can get there. If you don't want to write out your responses, that is okay. Try printing up these questions and placing them where you will see them every morning. Take a few minutes each day to reflect on them. Start walking through the field to make a new pathway!

Reflection Questions:

- Why do I want to learn how to meditate?
- What are my thought patterns that regularly get in the way of my happiness?
- What am I anxious about?
- What am I angry about?
- What makes me happy?
- What abundance do I have in my life right now?
- Is it hard for me to see this abundance?
- Do I get enough sleep?
- Do I feel tired all the time?
- Do I know what healthy eating means for me?

How will living a happy life bring even more joy to my life, and not only for me but for the ones I love and the community that surrounds me?

A Few Quick Basics about Meditation to Get You Started

In my life, I always strive for more knowledge. I believe that you are here to do the same. While this book is intended for beginners, I think that those with some experience can also gain new knowledge and inspiration from it.

It is important to follow some of the basic principles of meditation to achieve a useful practice. Your goal is to stop using your mind. Allow your body to achieve a state where you are at complete peace with yourself and your life in the moment. Here is some information to get you started.

If you have never meditated before, don't expect yourself to jump right into doing hours a day. You will not succeed. Give yourself time. Be kind to yourself. When you experience setbacks, don't beat yourself up. There is a reason meditating can be challenging, so let go and keep trying!

Environment

Setting up your environment for success is one of the best gifts you can give yourself. There are a lot of ways in which people don't get this right! A few easy steps:

- Do not sit in a room with a fan or air conditioning. Yes, you are meant to sweat! Often, after I meditate, I need to dry myself with a towel. So, have one handy for yourself as well.

- Make sure you will have no interruptions. If you are a beginner, you should always meditate indoors.

- Make sure there are no distractions, especially with sound.

Clothing

I often see people wearing tight yoga-style clothing when they meditate. This is not right. There is a reason why monks wear loose clothing. Your clothing should not restrict you. When it does, it stops the flow of your chi. Allowing chi to circulate freely through your body is important to your overall health. I will talk more about this concept in the next chapter. But for now, all you need to know is that you should wear loose fitting clothing.

Position and Posture

Sit cross-legged, with either one leg on top or both legs on top of each other. The second version may feel awkward at first because you are not used to it, but if it is something you'd like to try, don't let this stop you. Your body will get used to the position over time.

One very important aspect that I want to correct people on is the posture. So often, people sit with their backs straight when they should be leaning forward slightly. Lean forward just enough so that your backside is slightly higher. This posture is fundamental to allowing chi to flow.

Breath

When you breathe, you want to think about sending your breath to the dantian, located two inches below your navel. This is a Chinese term that essentially means your energy center, or center of power for the body. I will talk more about this in the next chapter. For now, as you take a breath in, place your hands just below your navel and imagine that breath traveling down to where your hands are. Try this a few times or until you feel your body understands the concept.

Meditation Breathing:

- Exhale to begin to get out all of the chi.
- Inhale deeply, pushing your chi down into your dantian. (Remember the feeling of your hands just below your navel.)
- When you inhale, hold your chi for 3 to 5 seconds.
- Exhale.
- Repeat this, 3 to 4 times.

Moving Forward

The peace I have searched for through all of the struggles I have faced in my life have led me here to you in this moment. I took my pain and made it my strength. If I hadn't faced those hardships, I may not have been inspired to develop the program that I have. Through meditation, getting a good night's sleep, and eating well, I pulled myself out of an unhealthy lifestyle filled with counterintuitive coping mechanisms to a happy life. I never believed that I could do this. After facing years of sadness, disappointment, and loss, I didn't think a happy, peaceful life was one I could achieve—until one day I knew my life would not be much longer unless I tried.

Let's walk forward together on your journey to getting happier and healthier!

Chapter 2

The Way of Meditation

"If you want to conquer the anxiety of life, live in the moment, live in the breath."
— Amit Ray

In this chapter, I will set you up to achieve success in your own meditation practice. As you already know, meditation has been life-changing for me. I know, with some dedication, it can do the same for you.

To begin your work, I'd like you to close your eyes once you've finished reading these instructions. When you do, open your mouth and exhale until you feel that you have nothing left to exhale. Then take one long, slow inhale and feel your breath moving all the way to your dantian. Remember that this is the place just below your navel.

Repeat this process 2 more times and, as you do, make a commitment to yourself. Commit to learning. Commit to growing. Commit to taking your health seriously. Commit to living a life of happiness!

A Healthy Smile

My husband and I regularly run a meditation class. One of the exercises we often do with our students is to take photos of their faces as they are meditating. This sounds strange, right? You might be wondering why we do this. Well, the answer is simple: Your face affects your mood. We want people to look at their facial expression while they are meditating because it is often very revealing. Most of our students have no idea they look the way they do. I often hear things like:

"I had no idea I look so angry."

Or,

"I look so sad."

Did you notice my face on the cover of this book? I didn't put it there to be vain or because I think I look nice. I put it there for two very specific reasons:

For you to feel the energy of meditation. There is a sense of calm in my posture that walks out of my meditation practice with me and into my daily life. This is what I want for you too.

My smile. Yes, your facial expression is very important!

There have been scientific studies that prove that when you smile you do feel happier. According to Fernando Marmolejo-Ramos: "In our research, we found that when you forcefully practice smiling, it stimulates the amygdala, which releases neurotransmitters to encourage an emotionally positive state."

I'm not saying you should pretend to be happy, or mask signs of depression or severe mental health issues. I'm not even saying you should suppress negative emotions by always having a smile on your face. What I am saying is that when you meditate, bring some awareness to your facial expression. Allow yourself to replace whatever is there with a soft smile, and see how it affects your mood in the moment.

If you find that this feels good to you, try smiling once in a while throughout your day. See how this feels. Does it help lift your mood? Does it help you find calm in moments when you need to slow your racing thoughts. Give it a try! If not anywhere else, do it in your meditation practice.

The Benefits of Meditation

Now that you are smiling and your spirit is ready, let's look a little closer at what we know meditation can do:

- Reduce stress
- Control anxiety
- Promote emotional health

- Increase self-awareness
- Improve concentration
- Slow aging

Wow! Don't all of these things sound amazing? Maybe it sounds too good to be true. Trust me, I have lived through some very stressful situations, as I shared with you in the first chapter, and have experienced much anxiety in my life; but since beginning my journey through meditation, I have learned how to control my own anxiety. I have increased my own selfawareness around what triggers me to feel angry, sad, worried, or stressed, and I have a greater ability to manage my emotions in these situations.

Life is stressful, but you can manage your response to it by learning how to focus on your breath rather than getting stuck living in your worried thoughts. With this sense of calm, you can reduce your negative responses to the stress and in turn bring more calm to your life.

By developing your ability to control your thoughts, effectively allowing you to stop living in them, you give yourself the gift of greater concentration as well. This is something I know our students feel great about. I work a lot with the older adult population and have heard often from my students how much more focus they have throughout the day, giving them a greater sense of accomplishment.

In our world, especially in the Western culture, many feel that life is over in the later years. You can't try anything new, in the same ways you did when you were younger. This is simply not true. When you have strong emotional health and an ability to focus on your goals, you can accomplish great things. Meditation has helped me learn this. And I think it is this belief, along with the great physical benefits of meditation, that has also helped me look at least 5 years younger than I did before I started meditating.

It is the truth! Looking younger has nothing to do with fancy creams or the latest beauty craze; it comes from within. When you feel younger, you look younger. When your organs are living in balance and working in harmony, it shows in your external appearance—not only in the reduction of wrinkles but also the way in which you walk out into the world. You walk with the strength and confidence of someone who has learned how to achieve balance within themselves.

Think about it this way: When you are tired, you walk differently than you do when you have energy. When your mind is clear of worry, you hold your head higher. You make eye contact with more ease. In a way, you physically, mentally, and emotionally say yes to living life in the moment—to being present. This way of being is noticeable in your physical presence.

As you continue to read this book, try bringing more awareness to your physical presence, in the same way that you are doing with your facial expression. How do you walk into the world? Do you hold your head high? Does your back feel slouched? Do your shoulders hold a lot of tension? You can write your reflections in a journal. That way, you can see you progress as you become more successful in your daily meditations.

There are so many benefits to meditating. I know from myself and my students that one of the big ones is sleeping through the night. When you sleep well, you feel better in every single aspect of your life.

Another benefit is having better circulation. I know a lot of people, as they age, complain more of having cold feet and cold hands. As you improve the flow of your chi, you will notice better circulation throughout your body, allowing your blood to warm up your cold extremities.

As you develop your own practice, you will begin to see these benefits within your own body and notice how they impact your overall health. You will feel younger, look younger, and have so much more energy!

Balancing Your Organs

One of the things that meditation does to help you look and feel better is to balance your organs. As a concept, the idea of balancing your organs might not be one that you've ever thought of before. It is one that is so important. All of your organs have an impact, not only on your emotional health but also on your physical and spiritual health.

Many people love to see fortune tellers to predict their futures and their entire lives. As for the Chinese, people love to read the yearly prediction book in relationship with their birth year, which in China has 12 zodiac elements according to the year of their birth.

For me, neither of these things are as important as the future your organs predict for you. I tell a lot of my friends that your future is your internal organs, which are your heart, liver, spleen, lungs and kidneys. If you have very healthy internal organs, that means you can eat, you can sleep, and you don't have any problems with your digestive system and your metabolism, which is the chemical reactions in the body's cells that change food into energy. Your body needs this energy to do everything from moving, to thinking, to growing.

Let's take a closer look at how we can live a healthier life by first balancing your five organs. Chinese medicine recognizes five elements:

- Fire
- Earth
- Metal
- Water
- Wood

These five elements are dynamic; they are always shifting and changing. Each element is connected to specific organs and emotions.

For example, wood is connected to both the liver and the gallbladder. The emotions that are associated with wood are anger, assertiveness, and kindness. If your anger is out of control, you can weaken your liver. Remember that everything is connected and shifting. You have the ability to shift yourself out of this state by recognizing it, understanding it, and moving beyond it.

The theories that have been developed regarding the five elements and how they interact within our bodies and our lives can be quite intricate. For the purpose of our work together, I am going to keep things simple. My goal for you is to be able to begin working within this concept right away, and to seek out more resources once you feel you have grasped what we do here together.

As I said, each organ is associated with one element. Here are the five we are going to focus on:

- Heart – Fire
- Liver – Wood

- Spleen – Earth
- Lung – Metal
- Kidney – Water

Each element is associated with specific emotions:

- Fire – Stress
- Wood – Anger
- Earth – Worry
- Metal – Grief
- Water – Fear

Therefore, the emotions that are associated with each organ are:

- Heart – Fire – Stress
- Liver – Wood – Anger
- Spleen – Earth – Worry
- Lung – Metal – Grief
- Kidney – Water – Fear

When each one of these is out of balance, it can affect your emotional health, your physical health, and your spiritual health.

Now, let's look at how emotions harm your body in relationship with your organs:

- Stress weakens your heart.
- Anger weakens your liver.
- Worry weakens your spleen.
- Grief weakens your lungs.
- Fear weakens your kidneys.

When we meditate, we achieve the goal of balancing these five organs. Through meditation, you improve your chi and your blood flow, which in turn nurtures your internal organs, and the organs act like a nonstop factory to support and give balance to your life. With a strong heart, you can overcome stress. With strong kidneys, you can fight your fear. With a strong liver, you can take control of your anger and respond from a place of calm. But there are so many more benefits to finding balance within your organs. For example, if your liver is good, your body will be more flexible. When your liver is in a healthy condition, then the tendons will be soft.

Meditation has the power to give strength to your body, to overcome the thoughts of the mind. One of the reasons we feel sick is because some organs begin to hold too much chi. When you focus on breathing into your dantian, sit in a good position, and give your mind a rest, you improve the flow of your chi and bring more balance.

Overcome Your Challenges

Everyone who builds a daily meditation practice will face challenges, especially in the beginning. If you've already begun, you probably know what I am talking about. Sometimes it can be helpful to join a class or even a discussion group. Get some support so that you don't give up!

One of the most common challenges I hear is:

"I can't do it!"

To which I say: "Of course you can; you just don't want to!"

When I see a student struggling with getting into their practice, I ask them to lie down and use the same breathing technique:

- Breathe all of the chi out.
- Breathe in and focus on sending the breath to the dantian.
- Breathe out.
- Repeat this 5 times.

My goal in doing this is to allow them to feel their chi throughout their entire body. Focusing on the chi can help your mind achieve calm.

Everyone has the ability to meditate if they make a commitment to trying. Yes, some days it will be hard to calm your mind. This is understandable. You face a lot in your daily life. Remember, you are strong! You can take control of your thoughts, your anxiety, your stress, and all the things that are making you feel tired, sad, angry, or sick.

You picked up this book because you are curious. You picked up this book because you know you want to feel better, and there is a part of you that understands that a healthy meditation practice is a big part of what you need right now. So, keep going. Lie down on a mat right now and practice feeling your chi.

Another common challenge most beginners face is achieving the posture. They find the numbness in their legs uncomfortable. This is also normal! That numbness, however, is a sign that you are healthy. Over time, you will get used to the posture and even come to enjoy it.

Sometimes beginners feel very sleepy when they meditate. This is also okay. You aren't used to being asked to sit for long periods of time and do nothing at all. In fact, life most often is the exact opposite. You are constantly being asked to get more done in a day than you have time for. Multi-tasking is applauded, while leaving work on time to create a positive work/life balance is looked down upon. Your body is constantly doing, while your brain is running ahead of it to prepare for the next task.

If you feel the need to sleep, let yourself sleep. In our class, we allow our students to sleep for 15 minutes if they feel the need to, and when we gently wake them up, we ask if they are ready to begin their practice.

Whatever challenges you face in your practice, know that you can always overcome them. If it feels like you can't, seek help! There is always someone out there who has been through similar moments to the ones you are experiencing.

Stop Using Your Mind, Start Using Your Breath

In the first chapter, I shared with you some simple ways to begin to set yourself up for a successful meditation practice. In this chapter, I want to share with you all you need to know to begin to understand the way of meditation.

Some of the points will be repetitive. This is okay. We learn by repetition. We learn by doing. To learn the way of meditation, you will not only learn how to breathe, but you will also learn how to prepare yourself and your space.

This is the way of meditation:

YOUR SCHEDULE

You should meditate at the same time every single day. Set an alarm for fifteen minutes as a beginner and add more time when you feel comfortable. It is your goal to sit 45 minutes for one sitting, for optimal healing benefits.

It is not as effective if you are meditating at different times of the day. It is also easier to find an excuse to let other tasks get in the way. This is why I advise people to meditate first thing in the morning. You are fresh. The events of the day are not yet pressing on your thoughts. Meditating is your biggest priority.

YOUR CLOTHING

Wear loose fitting clothing. This helps with the flow of your chi rather than cutting it off. I know those beautiful images of people wearing trendy yoga clothes looks inviting, but it is not appropriate to achieving good flow.

YOUR ENVIRONMENT

You need to set up a space for yourself indoors with no fan or air-conditioning. As you learned in Chapter 1, you are meant to sweat. Place a towel by your side for when you are done.

Make sure there are no loud noises. These can easily pull you out of your meditation, especially in the beginning. It is good to be able to close the door to the room you are in, so that you are not disrupted by family members or pets if you are meditating in your home.

Buy a good meditation cushion. This will help you achieve the proper posture.

YOUR POSTURE

- Use your meditation cushion to sit two inches higher than your legs when they are crossed.
- Put the weight of your body into your two knees. Your body should be leaning forward a bit.
- Relax your shoulders.

- Move your eyes to look out one foot away from your body. After you find that spot, keep your gaze on it for the duration of your warmup.
- Your head has to be straight; keep your chin a bit inward.
- Hold your two hands together in front of your legs. Place your left and right hand together with your two thumbs touching; hold them there in front of your legs. This is the way to perverse the chi of your body.
- Your legs should be crossed, either with only one on top or both ankles on top. When we don't cross our legs, 70% of our blood flow is in our lower body, from our waist to our toes. Once we cross our legs, the blood flow will be blocked and it will find a new way to flow, throughout the rest of the body. It is okay for your legs to feel numb after 15 or 30 minutes of meditating, or even sooner for some people. The numbness feeling is a sign that your body is healthy.

WARM UP

Do several exhales and inhales (exhale first, and then inhale and hold the breath for 3 to 5 seconds). Use your mouth to exhale and your nose to inhale; repeat that 5 times until you feel comfortable.

THE PRACTICE

After the above warm-up breathing technique, close your eyes.

If you are over 50 years old, close your mouth and roll your tongue. While meditating, you will have a lot of saliva; swallow the saliva slowly. The aim of this procedure is to activate and bring up the chi of your kidney, which is the water element. At the same time, this will activate and lower the chi of the heart, which is the fire element. Once the water and the fire meet, you will experience a greater sense of calm and will sleep better. This is the intercourse between heart and kidney, and the harmonization of the fire and water concept.

While meditating, keep your eyes closed. At the same time, open your internal eye and look forward through the middle of the forehead. While you are doing so, you have to be completely relaxed—do not put any force into it; do it naturally.

The internal eye is also called the third eye. The third eye is a mystical and esoteric invisible eye, usually depicted as located in the forehead, which provides perception beyond ordinary sight.

When you meditate, you have to close your eyes and then look forward through the center of your forehead. The technique asks you to be 100% relaxed and to look forward as if your eyes are open.

Once you close your eyes and look forward, you may have a lot of thoughts come into your mind.

As a beginner, it is hard to clear all the thoughts that you have while you are meditating. We have a technique called "Jue" (awareness) and "Zhao" (taking care of). What it means is that when you have a thought, you immediately allow yourself to become aware of the thought and then you take care of it by not going further into the thought.

Here is a real-life story to help you see what I mean:

After our class one day, I was talking with a member.

"Celia, I think I was able to use Jue and Zhao to help myself achieve a state of mindfulness meditation."

"Very good, Angela! How did you do this?"

"Without realizing it at first, I started to think about what to make for dinner tonight. Before I could start figuring out what I need to pick up on the way home and how to prepare it, in my mind, I stopped myself. I recognized that I was having the thought and I let it go."

"How did this time feel different than other times?"

"I felt strong. Normally my mind would have a hard time letting go. I'd have to let it get to the end of making a mental list of groceries and how I was going to make it, before I could stop thinking about it. And sometimes this thought process would loop again for fear I'd forget what I had decided. But this time, I told myself I'd figure it out after our session, and I let it go."

"Amazing work, Angela! How did the rest of your meditation go?"

"It went so well actually! More thoughts tried to come, and I used the

same techniques. I didn't get upset with myself or try to ignore the thoughts. Instead, I recognized them and let them know it was not the right time. I was able to let them go, and I came back to my meditation without frustration."

There is another technique, and we call it "Bai nian buru yinian," which means "a hundred thoughts are worse than a single thought."

This technique asks you to give yourself one thing to think about. My husband and I tell our class members to imagine a lotus flower. You close your eyes and then open the third eye to look forward, and you imagine that you see a lotus flower with your third eye. By holding this image in your mind, you put your concentration into one thought. When you generate enough chi from your dantian and your chi comes through the root chakra to the crown chakra, you will easily see the lotus flower with your third eye.

POST MEDITATION

Repeat the breathing. Exhale first with your mouth, and inhale with your nose for 5 times. Remember to do it slowly, softly, and smoothly.

Loosen your legs slowly. Then use your palms to slap the inside and outside of your thighs and your calves; on each side, do thirty-six slaps. The slapping is to get the blood flowing smoothly and to allow numbness to be released.

Stand up slowly.

THE RESULT

Once your chi and your blood flow improve, and your internal organs are in better health, we will awake feeling calmer, more beautiful, and refreshed.

Your Journey to Better Health

One of the analogies that I love is that of the numbers of your life. Zeros represent all the other areas of your life; for example, material wealth, your home, a good career, and the experiences you create for yourself and your loved ones.

The number one represents your health. Look at it this way:

0 – house
0 – career
0 – car
0 – travel
0 – hobbies
0 – other accomplishments

Without the 1, you have no wealth! Without your health, it is difficult to enjoy all the good in your life, even your family. Of course, they will still bring you joy and be there for you as best they can, but only you can give yourself the gift of good health.

Meditation is only the beginning, but it is a great place to start. I am so glad you have begun!

A Moment of Reflection

Now that you have begun your meditation practice, reflect on the following at least once a week:

- What challenges am I facing?
- How can I help myself get through these challenges?
- What successes am I feeling? (Keep in mind that these don't have to be monumental. They can be small, like: I meditated for ten full minutes before feeling sleepy. Or, I was able to quiet my negative thoughts for the full fifteen minute meditation this morning.) Recognize your wins and celebrate yourself for them.
- Have I noticed any improvements in my mental health? Or my physical health? (Again, these don't have to be big. Recognize every improvement you notice! This will help you see that you are progressing!)

CHAPTER 3
Healthy Mind, Healthy Body

"Learn to be calm and you will always be happy."

– Paramahansa Yogananda

Meditation brought me back to myself. It helped me to gain control over my sadness about past events in my life, my anxiety, and my worry for the future. It has also taught me how to live in the present moment. Every morning, I am grateful for another day. But mostly, I am grateful for this life and all the opportunities for growth that it has brought to me. This is the gift that meditation has given me: gratitude—gratitude for all that I have become.

Sitting quietly with myself has brought me the kind of inner peace that I always wanted but did not think was possible. I used to overthink about everything. It brought me much stress, and this brought me health problems. Stress is one of the worst things you can allow your body to experience. Stress not only causes premature aging, but it can also disrupt your sleep, cause stomach problems, bring on headaches, and bring tension to your relations. When I was able to recognize the things in life that were bringing me stress, and to then quiet my negative thoughts, I felt a vast improvement in my physical, emotional, and spiritual well-being.

In this chapter, I want to explore more of the benefits of developing a daily meditation practice. I have some stories to share with you to prove that meditation works. I have felt it and I have witnessed it.

Let Go of Stress

Over the years, I have had so many of our students report that they are better at managing their stress levels. Rather than living their days feeling worried, anxious, and depressed due to some of life's stressful situations, they instead release control and allow themselves to experience the good in life.

Think about how you feel when you are stressed about something. Maybe you have a new boss at work who is making things difficult for you. Every day, you worry about your career. This makes you irritable at home and more likely to lash out at your children, which in turn makes you feel bad about yourself. It becomes a vicious cycle of worry, anxiety, anger, and sadness, which can bring on a whole host of health issues and long-term depression.

When you meditate, you help yourself handle stress by taking a moment to breathe before reacting poorly. You allow yourself to think more clearly. Your body is stronger. You are able to clear your thoughts and make decisions from a productive place. Why?

Meditation does a few things to help you manage your stress:

It lowers your cortisol.

Cortisol is a hormone in your body that is released from your adrenal glands to help you manage stress. When your body's cortisol levels are constantly high, it has a negative impact on your body in many ways.

You can experience things like:

- Muscle weakness
- Severe fatigue
- Difficulty concentrating
- Acne
- Weight gain around the midsection
- High blood pressure
- Headaches

I think we can agree that living your daily life in a state of stress is detrimental both physically and emotionally. Take a moment to think about the stress you face daily in your life. Are you managing it? Does it feel like you are always stressed? Are you experiencing any of the negative symptoms listed above?

I want to share with you a story about one of our students whose meditation helped her release the stress in her life:

"Good evening, Susan. It's so nice to meet you."

"It's so nice to meet you too, Celia! I really hope you can help me."

"What is it you need help with?"

"I am so tired all day. I wake up tired and I go to bed tired. I am honestly tired of feeling tired."

Behind Susan's weak smile, I could feel her anxiety, her sadness, and her frustration. Because it was our first meeting, I did not want to pry too much into her life. I could feel in this moment that she needed some empathy and kindness.

"I believe we can help you, and I am so glad you are here. Why don't you come and find a spot in the room; I will show you how to find the proper posture."

At the end of our class, I could tell that Susan was disappointed. I knew that if she stuck it out, meditation could be life changing for her, and so I decided to check in with her.

"How are you feeling after that, Susan?"

"Honestly, I feel more frustrated. I couldn't stop the thoughts from coming, and the longer I sat, the worse they got. I think I feel worse."

"I am so sorry to hear that. But please, do not be disheartened. If meditating were easy, everyone would do it. There are so many benefits. I know I do not know you very well yet, but I do hope you will come back. Try this at home this week: For five minutes every day, find a quiet space and simply breathe in the way that we did at the beginning of the class. Focus on your breath. It is that simple. Do not be hard on yourself. Your goal is to help yourself feel better and not worse. It is normal to experience these challenges, especially in the beginning, but if you are able to stick it out, I promise it will help you feel more awake, focused, and energized."

Susan nodded. I knew she did not believe me, but I had some hope that she might give it another try.

She walked into our next class looking a little trepidatious.

"I am so glad you are back, Susan. Did you try the breathing exercise this week?"

"Thank you, Celia. I did, and it is the reason I am back. I can only do it at night before bed because the mornings are too busy for me, but I found that it helped to calm me before bed. I had such a good sleep the past two nights."

Over the following weeks, I got to know more about Susan and what was causing her exhaustion. One of the reasons Susan was so tired all day long was because she had to wake up very early in the morning to make breakfast for the whole family before going to work. After work, she then had to cook for the family again and do all the cleaning on her own so that the kitchen was ready for the next morning. To make matters more difficult, she lived with her mother-in-law, with whom she found it very difficult to communicate. She also shared with me that she sometimes felt it was difficult to communicate with her husband. Susan could not remember a time in her life when she did not live each day feeling stressed.

After two months of meditation, she told me that she was having an easier time communicating with her mother-in-law, which made her home life far less stressful. Her husband supported her meditation, which made her feel appreciated for the first time in a long time. Susan also shared with me that their relationship was also much better. She felt like she could ask him for help, and he would not get upset with her for it.

Susan had set up a time for about 30 minutes to meditate before she went to bed, on a daily basis, besides also coming to our meditation class once a week.

The quality of her sleep continued to become so much better, helping her feel more rejuvenated in the morning. She also found out that she had more energy and patience in the workplace. Susan also learned the importance of smiling; she discovered that she loved to smile at people. It made her feel good. People in the workplace and at home also responded to her differently when she smiled.

The reason for the changes Susan experienced was because her mindfulness meditation practice lowered the level of cortisol in her body. Reducing cortisol decreased the general stress, anxiety, and depression she was feeling. Susan was so much happier, and she loved to share her meditating experiences with all her friends. She began encouraging everyone she knew to meditate as well.

Meditation Break

- Sit cross-legged, with either one leg on top or both legs on top of each other, in a quiet, warm room. Set your alarm for 10 minutes.
- Exhale to begin to get out all of the chi.
- Inhale deeply, pushing your chi down into your dantian. (Remember the feeling of your hands just below your navel.)
- When you inhale, hold your chi for 3 to 5 seconds.
- Exhale.
- Repeat this, 3 to 4 times.
- Allow your mind and body to sit in silence. If you find unwanted thoughts getting in the way, always come back to your breath. Always be kind to yourself. Your thoughts can be powerful and they do not want to be silenced. Try not to get frustrated with yourself. Just calmly come back to your breath.

Listen to Your Body

"It is indeed a radical act of love just to sit down and be quiet for a time by yourself."
– Jon Kabat-Zinn

In the last chapter, I talked a lot about your organs, the elements they are connected to, and how you can use meditation to help bring them back into balance. The more tools you have available to you, the more you are able to listen to your body. Sitting quietly and simply listening is not only healing; it can also be revealing.

You, like me and most of humanity, live your daily life with a running dialogue going through your head. Some of it is useful and some of it is just noise. The noise can get in the way of so much information that your body is sharing with you. One of the greatest benefits of meditation is that it gives you the opportunity to check in with your body.

Many people report also beginning to eat better after developing their consistent meditation practice. This is not a coincidence. Have you ever gone through a very stressful time in your life, where you turned to food to feel better? We all do it. Your relationship with food can be a complicated one, but it really doesn't have to be. Your body knows exactly what it needs; it all becomes a matter of listening. But not only that, it is also about understanding what your relationship with food is.

Take a moment right now to think about your own eating habits. We are going to dive much deeper into this topic later in the book. I am introducing it now so that, as you continue developing your meditation practice, you can start to become more in tune with your body and understand how what you eat is affecting it.

Again, you can either record your responses or simply think about them as you answer the following questions:

- Do you allow your emotions to guide your eating habits?
- Do you eat more when you are upset, or do you eat less?
- If you were to rate yourself on your current daily eating habits, from 1 to 10 (10 being the most healthy, and 1 being the least), what number would you give yourself?
- How would your body benefit from eating more mindfully?

Another benefit of meditation is that it fosters a feeling of accountability to yourself. The more you become attuned to your body's needs, the more you want to do right by it. This self-awareness can help you develop strength in recognizing and dealing with addictions. If you know you drink too much alcohol, you are giving yourself a powerful tool to help yourself stop, or to get the help and support you need to heal your addiction.

A few more physical benefits to meditation are:

- Improved metabolism. Listening to your body and eating based on what you need rather than as an emotional response to your life's challenges, is one way your metabolism will improve. Also, meditation inspires people to move more. Again, you are able to hear the messages your body sends you. Often, when you do, it will tell you when it needs to be more active and when it needs to rest. When you are active, you help your body maintain a healthy metabolism, which in turn helps you keep the unwanted weight off!
- Improved digestion. We talked at the beginning of this chapter about stress and how meditation will help you regulate that stress. One of the negative impacts of stress on the body, along with all of the others, is its impact on your digestion. Stress can cause you to experience bloating, pain, and even troubles with your bowels. When you release your stress and work towards a more peaceful daily life, you help aid in your body's digestion.
- Meditation can help lessen chronic pain like arthritis. Living in pain can cause depression, stress, and anxiety. It becomes a vicious cycle of pain causing anxiety, and then that anxiety causing more pain. Meditation brings you out of that cycle. It allows you to release the anger and stress caused by the pain and to bring you to a place of calm. Within a place of calm, you have more strength in managing your condition.
- It can help you increase your sex drive. It all comes back to that mind-body connection again. When you listen to yourself and you feel good about yourself, you make better choices for your body. When you feel strength in yourself and confidence in your body, you give your sex drive a healthy boost. Consider it like filling the tank!
- When you are stressed, you cause inflammation throughout your body. That inflammation can cause a whole lot of different health conditions, such as diabetes and obesity, heart disease, and stroke.
- You look and feel younger! Reducing stress, eating well, and listening to your body will take years off your appearance.

Better than any facial cream or vitamin, it will relax the lines in your face. The confidence you feel within yourself will show in your posture. You will have more energy than you have had in years. Trust me! I work with a lot of older adults, and I have witnessed this in so many of them.

- It has been proven to be good for heart health and reducing blood pressure.

The list of physical benefits is so much longer. For now, I will stop here and share with you another story from one of my members:

"Celia, thank you so much for that session."

"You are so welcome. I am glad you are here."

"Me too. Have I told you yet about how much this class has helped?"

I had to stop for a moment and think. I was worried that she had told me and maybe I was not able to recall the memory in that moment.

"You know, Amy, I don't think so. Either way, I would love to hear it."

Amy's face lit up.

"When I first started, I was exhausted all the time. I knew why, but I didn't really think I could fix it. I used to have to get up almost every single hour in the night to go to the bathroom. I never woke up in the morning feeling rested because I never had a full night's sleep. I never could fall into a deep sleep because I was always having to get up again."

"Yes, actually, I think you told me this before coming to the class."

"Oh, yes… yes, it was you who told me meditation would help, and I have to be honest that I was skeptical, but you know what? It has done wonders. After only a month, I began sleeping straight through from 11 p.m. to 5 a.m. That's 6 whole hours of uninterrupted sleep. It's amazing. I feel so much better."

"I am so pleased! Thank you for sharing your story with me."

Let me explain to you why Amy experienced such a great result. When she meditates, her kidneys, which are the water element, go up, and her heart, which is the fire element, comes down, and this process creates the balance of the water and the fire: That is the heart and kidney interaction, which in turn improves the quality of her sleep, and she does not need to pee 5 times per night.

Meditation Helps with Your Emotions

"Meditation is choosing not to engage in the drama of the mind but elevating the mind to its highest potential."
— **Amit Ray**

I have talked about the benefits of meditation on stress, as well as the physical benefits of a regular practice. The last area I would like to focus on is your emotions. Your emotional response to your experiences can have a negative impact on your health and well-being, or a positive one.

Think about a time when you got really upset with someone you love because your emotions were so strong, you couldn't stop yourself. Maybe you yelled. Maybe it made your child cry or your wife not speak to you that night, or maybe your boss fired you. How did you feel after that?

Often, when we let our emotions get the better of us, we have a hard time seeing the reality of a situation and approaching it rationally from a calm frame of mind. We lash out. We overreact, and 99.99999% (maybe even 100%) of the time, we do not feel better for it. The situation is usually made worse rather than better. I have not met anyone in my lifetime who admits to never reacting emotionally to a hurtful situation. It happens to all of us.

Meditation can help you regain control in the heat of the moment. It can also help you control your thoughts when you are hurt or angry or upset.

Here are a few ways that can help you control your emotions:

- *When you meditate, you are retraining your brain so that when you are in a situation that is upsetting you, it automatically will switch to approach your response from a calmer place.*
- *When you meditate, you increase your serotonin, helping you stabilize your mood.*
- *When you meditate, you are more relaxed. As I previously talked about, it lowers your blood pressure, helping you stay grounded in tough situations.*

- *When you meditate, you are essentially teaching yourself to calm yourself without relying on outside stimulants such as alcohol or drugs.*
- *When you meditate, you are giving your brain a break. Essentially, you're allowing your brain to not burn out. In this time of rest, it gains more strength.*
- *When you meditate, you teach yourself how to focus on your breath. This is an incredible tool to use when needing to calm your emotions in the moment.*
- *When you meditate, you are showing yourself how much you value and love yourself. When you feel loved, it is easier to be more compassionate towards others.*

Meditation is life-changing when it comes to your communication skills and your ability to control your emotions in the moment. I am going to share one last success story with you for this chapter:

Freddie walked into class and I could tell immediately he was feeling low. I smiled at him and decided to let him come and talk to me if he needed to. I felt like he was not ready to talk about it yet.

During our class, I noticed him open his eyes at one point and rub his forehead. He needed some guidance. I walked over to him and spoke quietly:

"Freddie, I know you are here because you have some very important goals to achieve."

He nodded, looking tearful.

"Come back to your breath. Do not complicate it. Just breathe. Remember to breathe out fully, and when you breathe in, focus on sending that breath to your dantian."

At the end of the session, Freddie was the last one to stand up. He was ready to talk. He had only been coming for a month, but I knew him well enough to know that he would not approach me.

I walked over to him and asked, "Did the reminder to breathe help?"

"Honestly, Celia, I don't know. I appreciate you trying to help, but I may be a lost cause."

"You are not a lost cause! Remind me why you came."

Freddie took a deep breath in and met my eyes. "Because I get so mad all of the time. I yell at my wife and kids and my colleagues. It never feels good. I feel like everyone tip toes around me and I hate that. Sometimes I don't even know why I'm so mad; or the reason I'm so mad is so small, it shouldn't even matter."

"Did something happen since our last class?"

He seemed reluctant to respond. I waited and he finally did.

"Yeah. I yelled at one of my new employees in front of everyone yesterday. It was over something so stupid. He had forgotten to prepare a short document for our team meeting that day. It wasn't anything that really mattered, and it could've been emailed after the meeting. Anyway, this morning, the whole team was quiet. I asked them why, and one very brave employee told me they had had enough of my temper. I say "brave" because she looked terrified. That is what hurt. I don't want to terrify people. I thought I was doing better but obviously I'm not."

"First of all, it takes time, so be patient and kind with yourself. Once you can do that, you can also do the same with others. It is through self love that you will achieve success. Next time you feel like your emotions might get the better of you, remember what I just did in the session. Can you tell me?"

"Yes, you reminded me to focus on my breath."

"Yes. If it does not work right away, do not get angry with yourself. Try again. If you are in a situation where this does not feel comfortable for you, simply tell the person or people you are with that you need a moment. Find a quiet place and remember to exhale for long enough to expel the chi, and then send your inhalation to your dantian."

"I will keep working."

"I am so glad. I know you can achieve your goals. Stay the course."

It took Freddie six months of coming to our class to feel that he had achieved success in his goals. When he came across difficult people and situations, he immediately took a deep breath and stopped using his mind. Basically, he sent a signal to himself to stop thinking, by concentrating on taking deep breaths for 3 to 5 seconds. By doing so, he didn't react to the difficult people or the situations impulsively. When he meditated, he trained his brain to focus on the present, and this helped him learn to control and process his emotions in the moment. Once he stopped using his mind for just a few seconds, he turned his focus toward his breath, which created a kind of relief in his mind.

A Moment of Reflection

Think about the three stories I shared with you in this chapter and reflect on the following:

Thinking towards the future, what would your meditation success story be. How would quieting your mind help you achieve your physical, emotional, and even spiritual goals?

If you feel called to, write out a story in the same way that I did the ones here. You can be talking to a teacher or a friend or a loved one and telling them all about your success and how much it means to you!

Chapter 4

The Importance of Sleep

"The best bridge between despair and hope is a good night's sleep."
– E. Joseph Cossman

One of the best things you can do for yourself is to get a good night's sleep. While you may not feel it, there is so much good that happens within your body while you sleep. In this chapter, I will share with you some of the ways in which you can help yourself get a better night's sleep, how a good night's sleep will help with your meditation practice, and also how meditation helps you to achieve better sleep habits.

The Best Time of Night to Sleep

Did you know that there is an optimal time of night to sleep? You may have said or heard someone say: "I am a night owl. I can't fall asleep before 1 or 2 a.m."

Well, it may feel right, but you could be doing your body a disservice. I always share with people that the best time to sleep at night to get enough energy the next day is to go to bed before, or at the very latest, 11 p.m. This is when your body can achieve optimal rest and rejuvenation.

According to *The Yellow Emperor's Classic of Internal Medicine*, "When yang qi in one's body has been used up, one should lie down, and when the yin qi has been used up, one needs to sleep. During 11 p.m. to 1 a.m., and 11 a.m. to 1 p.m., the yin qi and the yang qi are alternating, so it is the best time to actually go to bed and rest.

Midnight is when yin qi and yang qi—water and fire, respectively—meet. This is called *Heyin* or "yang joining with yin." It is at this point where yin qi is at its strongest. At noon, the opposite occurs; yang qi is at its strongest and is when "yin joins with yang," also known as *Heyang*.

Yang qi in the human body is like the sun in nature. It is recorded in the *The Yellow Emperor's Classic of Internal Medicine* that there are 24 solar terms in a year and 24 solar terms in a day. Five o'clock in the morning is equivalent to the solar term "Awakening of the Insects" (jīng zhé), which is also when the sun starts to rise. It is therefore best to awaken at this time. When our body's energy resonates with the energy of the universe and the energy of nature, we enhance our body's energy.

I am going to share a table here to show you what you should do during the 24-hour qi cycle in order to better manage your health.

Follow the Time to Stay Healthy

Certain organs function optimally at certain times of the day. The organs act as the biological clock hidden in the body, and if you listen, you will begin to feel it. These are the times of day when you should rest, sleep, eat, drink, and try to have a bowel movement:

- 5 a.m. to 7 a.m. – Large intestine is on duty (toilet).
- 7 a.m. to 9 a.m. – Stomach is on duty (breakfast).
- 9 a.m. to 11 a.m. – Spleen is on duty (stretch).
- 11 a.m. to 1 p.m. – Heart is on duty (rest).
- 1 p.m. to 3 p.m. – Small intestine is on duty (lunch).
- 3 p.m. to 5 p.m. – Bladder is on duty (drink water).
- 5 p.m. to 7 p.m. – Kidney is on duty (dinner).
- 7 p.m. to 11 p.m. – Cardiac meridian and triple energizer meridian are on duty (rest & meditate).
- 11 p.m. to 5 a.m. – Gall bladder, liver, and lung are on duty (sleep).

If someone wants to nap at a different time in the day, they should follow the needs of their body and take a nap right away, because our practice is to follow the needs of our body and to listen to the internal voice of our needs. Take a 15 to 30-minute nap if you need to, and it will eventually help you to regulate your internal clock to achieve the goal of maintaining a healthy body and mind.

Also, if you have a lot of things to do and you think that you are going to stay up late at night to get them all done, the best thing to do is to go to bed before or at 11 p.m. and sleep until 1 a.m., and then get up again to finish what you need to do.

If you are one of those people who have a hard time falling sleep early at night, my suggestion for you is to try to get up really early in the morning. This way, you will be tired earlier. Keep trying to get up early until this habit is shifted.

Get Up Early

Many people get up early because they feel they can get more done in the morning. This is true, but the most beneficial reasons for getting up early, in addition to accomplishing more in a day, has more to do with your physical health and overall well-being.

Consider your body to be its own small universe, with the yin and yang energy flowing within: Within one day, your liver represents the spring time in the morning; at noon, your heart is the summer time; in the evening, your lungs represent the fall; and at night, your kidneys are the winter. When you can experience the full four seasons in your body within a day, your organs are living in balance with the cosmic energy of the universe. When you awake with the sun, you help your body achieve this balance by aligning your energy with that of the cosmic energy.

If you want to know whether your organs are in balance, you have to bring all your organs into balance. Your digestive system and also your spleen and stomach support all the organs, which means that if your organs are imbalanced, the first thing to adjust is your digestive system so that your body is nurtured with nutrients.

During a 24-hour period, your energy/qi moves through the organ systems in two-hour intervals. Qi draws inward to help restore the body between the hours of 1 a.m. and 3 a.m. The liver cleanses the blood and performs other functions, such as getting the blood ready to travel outward into the rest of the body.

Over the next 12 hours, qi cycles through the organs that assimilate, digest, and eliminate food through the body or our diurnal organs. By mid-afternoon, the body begins to slow down again in preparation for the nocturnal phase.

The nocturnal phase is all about restoring and maintaining. So, when one organ system is at its peak, its counterpart, on the opposite side of the clock, is at its lowest point. Here is an example of what I mean:

Between 7 a.m. and 9 a.m. are the hours of the stomach. This is when the stomach is at its peak, and also why it is recommended to eat a big breakfast. On the opposite side of the clock lies the pericardium, which is associated with the pituitary, hypothalamus, and reproductive organs. The pericardium is at its weakest point between the hours of 7 a.m. and 9 a.m.

Achieve Balance in Your Body

Do you wake up every night or every morning about the same time? Have you ever wondered why? Some people call that an internal clock. However, Chinese medicine gives a much deeper look into how the body functions.

Chinese medical theory divides the body based upon the 12 energetic meridians. Each of the meridians is assigned a two-hour time slot. For example, the liver meridian is associated with the hours of 1 a.m. to 3 a.m. If you wake up during this time frame, then there is an issue with your liver meridian. Knowing this information can be very important in order for us to manage our health.

Let's take a look back at the table I shared above and think about it again. I've summarized it a bit differently to get you thinking about it on a higher level. Think about it in terms of creating an overall balance in your body.

It is, again, a brief summary of the 24-hour qi cycle:

- 3 a.m. to 5 a.m. is lung time.
- 5 a.m. to 7 a.m. is large intestine time.
- 7 a.m. to 9 a.m. is stomach time.
- 9 a.m. to 11 a.m. is spleen time.
- 11 a.m. to 1 p.m. is heart time.

- 1 p.m. to 3 p.m. is small intestine time.
- 3 p.m. to 5 p.m. is urinary bladder time.
- 5 p.m. to 7 p.m. is kidney time.
- 7 p.m. to 9 p.m. is pericardium time.
- 9 p.m. to 11 p.m. is triple burner time (associated with the thyroid and adrenals)
- 11 p.m. to 1 a.m. is gall bladder time.
- 1 a.m. to 3 a.m. is liver time.

If you have recurring problems at the same time every day, then there is a good chance that the organ/meridian associated with that time is in distress. This is why traditional Chinese medicine practitioners ask so many questions, and also why they look at the body as a whole instead of just at one particular organ. By understanding that every organ/energetic meridian has a maintenance schedule to keep daily, you can then treat your body properly so that you achieve the ultimate health and well-being.

What will happen to your health if you don't have enough sleep?

Conventional wisdom says that the average adult should aim to get about eight hours of sleep each night. The fact that you become tired and need to sleep at times proves that this is vital to the body's functioning. Just as you need to eat, drink a certain amount of water, and exercise to stay healthy, you also need to get a good night's sleep.

Do you prioritize your sleep? If you are like many people, it is the last thing on your list. An average person gets less than six hours of solid sleep each night. If you are the average person, you are sleep deprived. Make a commitment to yourself to start getting eight hours of sleep. Your body needs this rest to recoup energy expended during the day. A serious lack of sleep weakens the immune system to increase the likelihood of infection.

Tips to Sleep Well

"The minute anyone's getting anxious, I say, 'You must eat and you must sleep. They're the two vital elements for a healthy life.'"
— Francesca Annis

- **Stay active.**

Daily exercise often helps people sleep. I like to walk to the mountain in the morning at 6 a.m., for an hour. Since I started doing this, I have noticed that I automatically get very tired around 10:30 p.m. I go to bed at this time and fall asleep very easily.

When choosing the type of exercise you want to do each day, choose something that you like doing so that it doesn't feel like a chore that you can easily talk yourself out of. I choose this morning walk because it is beautiful. I love looking out at the nature that surrounds me. Each morning, I am happy to take this walk. What do you love to do? If you haven't found it yet, try new things. Maybe try taking a morning swim at your local community center, or a dance class. There are so many ways to stay active; you might as well have fun doing it!

- **Maintain a healthy sleep environment.**

Control your room temperature. Extreme temperature may disrupt your sleep. The discomfort of being too hot or too cold will wake you up constantly throughout the night.

Tidy your room before you sleep, and you will wake up the next day with a pleasant feeling. Living in a cluttered space can affect your thoughts subconsciously. Keep your space organized and you will also feel more organized within your own thoughts.

Turn off your cell phone and computer. People usually worry that they will miss a call when they sleep. If that is your situation, remember that your health is very important to you. Getting a good night's sleep is as important as having a successful business. Therefore, I always mention to my friends that in order to have good health, you have to have good sleep, and that means you will have a good today and a good future.

- **Avoid drinks or foods that contain caffeine or alcohol.**

Caffeine is found in coffee, nonherbal teas, soda, and chocolate, and acts as a stimulant that can keep you awake. My body reacts to caffeine strongly, so I have to avoid drinking tea and coffee after 12 noon. If you have a body like mine, you may need to avoid drinks or foods that contain caffeine as well.

Alcohol prevents people from entering deep sleep, which is necessary for physical and emotional restoration.

- **Plan a bedtime routine.**

Your sleep will benefit greatly when you have a plan in place to deescalate from your day. Human beings are creatures of habit, and by setting a routine into motion, we are alerting our brain that it is time to sleep.

Before you go to bed, you can take a warm bath or shower and listen to light music. My way of getting a good night's sleep is to meditate for 30 minutes before I go to bed. You may be creative and create your own habits. Yet, it is very important that you give yourself enough down time between working on your computer or answering calls or texts. All these will stimulate your brain and make it hard to fall asleep.

- **Meditation helps you sleep.**

Meditation slows down your heart rate and lowers the level of the stress hormone, cortisol, in your body, two things that happen naturally when you sleep. Meditation can help you to achieve the brainwaves of the same state your brain enters when you are falling asleep.

If chronic pain keeps you awake at night, developing a meditation practice can help. If you find it is your anxious thoughts that are keeping your brain from allowing you to fall asleep easily, meditation can also help to break these thought patterns.

Meditation Skills to Help You Sleep

Whether you have regular insomnia or you just need some help adjusting to a new sleep schedule, meditation before sleep may have benefits.

- Let go of your thoughts. Meditation is all about letting go of judgment. Thoughts may come into your head as you try to relax. Simply observe them without judgment. Notice them and allow them to fade away as you focus on your meditation.
- Breathe! Breathe out first and count for 3 to 5 seconds; then breathe in and hold the qi for 3 to 5 seconds again.
- Listen to calming sounds. Some people enjoy meditating while listening to calming music or natural sounds like rain or ocean waves. Find one that you like and try it out. It will help you to relax and then sleep better.
- Relax your body. It is very important to listen to your internal voice and relax your body. Drop your shoulders and smile before allowing the muscles in your face to relax.

Once you get used to the routine of meditating for ten to thirty minutes daily before bed, you will see great results immediately.

Sleep Helps You Meditate

Once you begin to practice daily, you will also notice that when you are rested, you will also find it easier to meditate. They work together to help you achieve calm, strength, and peace. It is certain that if you have a good night's sleep, especially following the 24-hour qi cycle, it will help you develop a beneficial meditation practice. When you have enough sleep, you can meditate better. You will then receive all the benefits of meditation.

Case Study

Susana was a business woman for over thirty years. During that time, the stress of her work caused her to develop chronic insomnia. She needed to take sleeping pills to sleep.

"You know, Celia, it is so strange. I am now retired, and the worries

of my business no longer haunt my thoughts, but I still can't sleep. I really thought that without the stress, my insomnia would go away."

"I'm sorry to hear this, Susana. But it really isn't that surprising. Humans are creatures of habit. You developed a life-long habit of relying on pills to help you calm yourself before bed. For years now, I imagine that is just what your body has gotten used to, and so it is this rather than the stress that is getting in the way of your sleep."

Susana seemed to be pondering what I just said, and I could tell she did not believe me. Of course, if you have spent years believing that you need a pill to sleep because you are stressed, it is difficult to hear someone tell you that you might have been the person to create the habit that was the cause of your current problem.

"Why don't you give our meditation class a try. You don't have to stay if you find it doesn't work for you, but I have seen meditation help so many people overcome years of chronic insomnia and begin sleeping without the aid of drugs for the first time in years."

"You know what, I am going to give it a try. I am so tired of feeling tired. And while the drugs do help me sleep, I never really feel rested."

I spoke with Susana after a month of coming to our class.

"How are you, Susana? My husband told me that you reported to him that you were sleeping better."

"You were right! I needed some tools to help me break a habit of relying on drugs to calm my stress."

"I am so happy to hear this! Which tools have helped you the most?"

"The first one is breathing. Practicing deep breathing helps me both relax into my meditation practice and into sleep at night."

"Yes!"

"Also, I realized that it wasn't just my thoughts that were wound up but my body too. Of course, it is all connected. I just never really put it together before. Meditation has helped me learn how to feel where the tension is in my body and how to relax it. But I think that one of my most important realizations is that I was often stressed about nothing. My mind was still thinking that I have a lot of burdens, when much of these have been eased since retirement."

"Good. Have you been able to overcome this feeling?"

"Mostly, yes. Some days the old thoughts creep in, and when they do, I try to do what you taught me. I do my best to recognize the thoughts and then to let them go."

"When thoughts enter your mind, don't be nervous; it is very normal for you to have thoughts in your mind. Just observe them and don't give any judgements, and don't follow the thoughts to create more thoughts," I reminded her.

"Thank you! Yes, I have to tell you that your lessons have helped so much. Breathing, relaxing my body, and letting go of my nagging thoughts, have helped me to both meditate and sleep."

When Susana first took our class, she couldn't sit for fifteen minutes. Eventually, after two months of practicing, she could meditate for 30 minutes on her own before she went to bed at night. She came back to me and told me that she finally didn't need to take sleeping pills, and she could manage to sleep five to six hours without getting up in the middle of the night. And she listened to my advice to go to bed at or before 11 p.m. She also turned off her cell phone and TV one hour before bed.

A Moment of Reflection

Take some time to think about your sleep habits. Reflect on the following questions:

- Do you regularly get a healthy night's sleep?
- If not, what is getting in the way?
- How can you change your habits to help yourself have a better night's sleep?
- Are you getting enough exercise in the day?
- If not, what is stopping you from being active?
- What types of exercise do you enjoy the most?

Chapter 5

The Color of Food

"If you are planning for a year, sow rice; if you are planning for a decade, plant trees; if you are planning for a lifetime, educate people."

(Chinese Proverb)

When my son was young, he loved the color blue. One day I decided to paint his bedroom blue for him. When I brought him in to see it, he was so happy.

"Oh, Mom, I like it a lot. I feel very comfortable and calm."

Everyone has a color that they love. It may make them feel calm, like blue does for my son, or it may make them feel joy, like a bright orange-yellow does for my older sister.

In Chinese culture, color holds a higher significance. Each color is also tied to an element. For example, red is fire, white is metal, yellow is earth, and black, although not always seen as a lucky color, is water. Green represents the wood element and symbolizes spring. The Chinese pay a lot of attention to color.

During Chinese New Year, people love to wear red clothes. Red is a popular color in Chinese culture, symbolizing luck, joy, and happiness. It also represents celebration, vitality, and fertility in traditional Chinese color symbolism. Red is the traditional color worn by Chinese brides, as it is believed to ward off evil.

Pink is regarded as a shade of red, and so it is also believed to bring good fortune and joy. Green in Chinese culture symbolizes cleanliness, eco-friendliness, harmony, and growth. Yellow is believed to bring good luck, which is why you will often see it paired with red.

Western culture also pays a lot of attention to color but attaches their own beliefs and symbolism. Why is red associated with Valentine's Day? Because it is a symbol of the heart, of love. But red also means stop. Stop lights are red. Stop signs are red. Often, warning signs are also in red. Teachers often grade (used to anyway) papers in red ink.

Everywhere in the world, people associate certain events, emotions, and objects with color. Why do we associate colors with certain events, emotions, or objects? In traditional Chinese medicine, color association is all about the theory of the five elements. This theory also extends to the foods that we eat.

The color associations linked to the physical and emotional characteristics in the five elements theory, are relationships between things that should start us thinking on a deeper level about connections. The more connections we make between the outside and the inside worlds, the deeper our understanding of ourselves as part of the bigger picture of nature becomes.

The Five Elements in Chinese Cuisine

Chinese herbalists and doctors believe that to properly treat a patient, you must know the state of the five elements in their body. Any deficiency or an excess of an element can lead to illness.

As I have already talked about, the five elements also represent our five main organs:

- Lung – Metal
- Liver – Wood
- Kidney – Water
- Heart – Fire
- Spleen – Earth

As I just shared with you, the five elements also represent five colors:

- White – Metal
- Green – Wood
- Black – Water

- Red – Fire
- Yellow – Earth

Here is a table to show your emotional feelings and your tastes, in relationship with the five organs, the five elements, and the five colors:

Element	Organ	Color	Feeling	Taste
Wood	Liver	Green	Rage	Sour
Fire	Heart	Red	Happiness	Bitter
Earth	Spleen	Yellow	Thought	Sweet
Metal	Lung	White	Sorrow	Spicy
Water	Kidney	Black	Fear	Salty

How do emotions harm your body?

- Grief weakens your lungs.
- Worry weakens your spleen.
- Stress/excessive happiness weakens your heart. (One sample of this is when some people suddenly hear great news and have a heart attack in the next second. It is because their heart couldn't support the sudden change of the mood.)
- Fear weakens your kidneys.
- Anger weakens your liver. (When your liver is damaged, your mood will be affected, and you will get angry more often. One example of this is when you don't have enough sleep; it will affect your liver and you may have a shorter temper.)
- Eating sour food will enhance the function of your liver.
- Bitter food supports your heart.
- Sweet food supports your spleen.
- Spicy food supports your lungs.
- Salty food supports your kidneys.

However, everything has to be balanced. You shouldn't consume too much of any one taste. My uncle loved to eat very salty food. He didn't control himself, and my aunt always complained that he used too much salt when he cooked. He put soy sauce on all food, even if it was salty already. Eventually, he had kidney stones and he died from kidney cancer.

Use 5 Color Rules for Your Diet

In Chinese culture, food and medicine are closely related. There is a saying: "If you want to have good health, nurturing your body in daily life with good diet is better than taking medicine."

To help show you what I mean, I want to share with you a story from the old days in China:

There were two brothers who lived in a big city. The younger brother was a very famous doctor. All of the patients who came to see the younger brother were cured. They all talked about what a wonderful doctor he was.

One day one of his patients said to him: "You are the best doctor we have in this city."

"I am actually not a good doctor," he replied.

His patient looked very puzzled.

"What do you mean? You have helped me feel better. You helped cure my cousin, and you helped my mother manage her chronic pain. You have healed everyone I know who has come to see you. I have not heard of any other doctor with as high a success rate as you."

"That is because you have not heard of my older brother."

"If I have not heard of him, then he must not be better than you."

"I can assure you that he is."

"Why have I not heard of him then?"

"Because my elder brother cures people before they get sick. He has ways to help people stay healthy. Yet, I cure people after they get sick. Which one do you like better?"

You get to make a choice every single day with the food you eat. Do you want to stay healthy by preventing illness before it starts, or would you rather rely on modern medicine to fix the problem after it's already begun. I do not know about you, but I would rather not encounter the health issue at all! The bottom line is that having a good diet prevents illness! You become what you eat!

According to *The Yellow Emperor's Classic of Internal Medicine,* you can achieve a healthy body by consuming food with five colors and five tastes. This simple principle is also becoming more understood in the Western world as well. This brief quote comes from the Harvard Medical School:

"My response is simple: Eat all of the colors of the rainbow," says Dr. Michelle Hauser, a clinical fellow in medicine at Harvard Medical School and a certified chef and nutrition educator. "These colors signal the presence of diverse phytochemicals and phytonutrients."

"Phytochemicals and phytonutrients are beneficial substances produced by plants. People who eat diets rich in phytonutrients have lower rates of heart disease and cancer—the two leading causes of death in the United States."[1]

To understand more about how colorful foods help each organ of the body, see the list on the next page, of how the color groups provide benefits for the corresponding organs.

- **Liver** – Green food enhances the function of our liver.
- **Heart** – Red food enhances the function of our heart.
- **Spleen** – Yellow food enhances the function of our spleen (the digestive system).
- **Lungs** – White food enhances the function of our lungs.
- **Kidneys** – Black food enhances the function of our kidneys.

Green Food

There are all kinds of green vegetables, and green grapes! Green vegetables deliver omega-3 fatty acids, vitamin K, folic acid, and more good things, with very few calories.

Green is the color associated with the liver in Chinese medicine; and if your liver is weak, you should eat a lot of green food to enhance the function of the liver. If you get angry easily, you should put a lot of green vegetables into your diet to balance your organs.

---

[1] https://www.health.harvard.edu/staying-healthy/add-color-to-your-diet-for-good-nutrition

Sample meal for your liver (Green)

Cucumber & Quail Meat

Ingredients

100 grams of quail meat
100 grams of winter bamboo shoots
5 grams of mushrooms
15 grams of cucumbers
Half an egg white
Starch

Directions

First slice the quail meat.
Mix the quail meat with egg white and starch.
Stir fry; then add winter bamboo shoots, mushrooms, and cucumbers, and fry until cooked.

Red Food

Some examples of red food are cherries, tomatoes, and beets. Red foods are high in two phytochemicals: lycopene and anthocyanins. These are good for your heart. And not only that, they also lower your risk for certain cancers.

Red food supports your heart, and your heart, in mood, is happiness. It is also the strongest of all the colors in evoking emotion. If we have a healthy heart, we will be happier. In Chinese medicine, both the heart and the brain are called the heart. The heart dominates the blood vessels and occupies the most important position in the organs.

Sample meals for the heart (Red)

Number 1

A bowl of porridge a day keeps the doctor away! It nourishes the heart, nourishes the spleen, nourishes the qi, and nourishes the blood. It soothes the mind and clears the heart!

If you feel like you cannot sleep, experience forgetfulness, wake up suddenly at night, are dreamy, experience neurasthenia (chronic fatigue), or feel unable to eat, you must make this bowl of porridge!

Eight Treasures Nourishing Heart Porridge!

Ingredients:

Codonopsis
Longan
Jujube
Lily
Chinese yam
White lentils
Coix seed
Lotus seeds
Japonica rice

Directions:

Soak lotus seeds, Chinese yam, lily, and coix seed in water for 15 minutes.
Remove the core of the jujube.
Put the codonopsis slices into the pot, together with the japonica rice and longan meat, and add an appropriate amount of water.
First boil with high heat; then switch to low heat and cook until the porridge is thick.
Add rock sugar and cook for a while before eating. It's really simple!

Originally, this recipe called for ginseng, but I changed it to codonopsis for everyone. After all, ginseng is still relatively expensive. For daily supplements, codonopsis is enough!

Number 2

Red cabbage is rich in calcium, phosphorus, iron, carotene, vitamin C, and other ingredients, which not only help the body improve resistance, but also maintain the normal metabolism of human tissues and cell structures.

Stir-Fried Red Cabbage Heart

Ingredients

Red cabbage heart
Oil
Garlic
Salt

Directions

Pick the vegetables first. I picked each 8CM as a section.
Wash the vegetables.
Heat oil in a pan; add garlic (popping flat).
Stir fry for 4 minutes.
Add salt to taste.

Yellow Food

Some great examples of yellow foods are orange peppers, yellow peppers, pineapple, pumpkin, and corn. Yellow foods are high in Vitamin C, which enhances the function of your spleen. According to Chinese medicine, the functioning of the spleen impacts our digestive system. The spleen transforms and transports the energy from the food you eat, throughout your body.

Yellow foods have unique health properties that ward off oxidative stress, promote gut health, and support a balanced microbiome. When your gut is not working optimally, it can take a toll on the whole body, and the bacteria inside it. Yellow foods modulate the secretion and activity of enzymes that help break down your food and participate in the natural detoxification processes of the body.

Sample meal for your spleen (Yellow)

Pumpkin Porridge

It warms the heart and nourishes the stomach! It is really fragrant. People who have no appetite can't help but eat two more bowls when they see this bright color and experience the delicate flavor.

Ingredients

Pumpkin (preferably an old pumpkin; the older, the sweeter)
Corn kernels (I do not use fresh corn. The porridge made from dried corn is also delicious.)
Rice

Directions

Soak corn kernels and rice for half an hour, so that the porridge is more delicious.
Shred the pumpkin.
Put the pumpkin in the pot and steam for about fifteen minutes.
Take another pot; put the rice in the pot and cook it first.
After the rice is cooked for 25 minutes, add the corn kernels, stir well, and continue to cook for about five or six minutes.
Finally, put in the pumpkin puree. It will be done in five or six minutes.

White Food

Delicious examples of white foods are lotus root, turnip, onion, garlic, pear, almond, white sesame, white mushroom, cauliflower, white leek, honeydew melon, and parsnip.

If your lungs are feeling weak, or you know that you are experiencing health issues with your lungs, help yourself breathe easier by including more white foods in your diet!

Sample meal for your lungs (White)

Ginseng Pork Ribs Soup

Ingredients

Pork ribs
Yam
Wolfberry
Polygonatum odoratum
Ginseng
Candied dates
1 slice ginger
Salt to taste

Directions

The ribs first fly into the water; that is, put water and ribs in the pot, and then pick up the ribs after boiling.
Put the spareribs together with Chinese yam, wolfberry, ginseng, candied dates, and ginger in a pot; add boiling water and cook together. After the soup boils, reduce the heat and simmer for more than an hour. After cooking, add some salt to taste.

Black Foods

If I were to ask you to think of some foods that you would consider to be black right now, what would you say? Can you think of any? I know! This is a harder one. How about these black foods: black mushroom, sea cucumber, black sesame, and black rice. Help your kidneys reach their full potential and achieve optimal functioning by adding some of these black foods, and any others you may have thought of, to your diet.

Sample meals for the kidneys (Black)

Purple Rice Porridge

This delicious recipe will nourish your kidneys, invigorate your spleen, and warm your liver, as well as improve your eyesight and invigorate your blood.

Ingredients

Black rice
Brown rice
Mulberry
Purple rice
Blueberry jam

Directions

Wash the mulberries.
Soak them in salt water for 30 minutes.
Dry the mulberries.
Add purple rice, black rice, and brown rice to the pot, and cook into porridge. Add mulberries and continue to cook for 10 minutes.
According to personal taste, add blueberry jam for seasoning.

Listen to Your Body

I eat a lot of the black food myself because I was born with a weak kidney. Although Hawaii does not have winter, when it comes to Christmas and Chinese New Year, I will make black rice, black sesame seed cake, and black fungus soup with chicken.

Winter is the season of nourishing the kidneys. The nutrients in winter can be absorbed and stored in the kidneys. In addition to proper exercise to benefit the kidneys, diet is so important. In particular, foods such as black rice, black beans, black sesame seeds, and black fungus are good products to nourish the kidneys.

Kidney governs water, stores essence, and is the foundation of the innate, which means with insufficient endowment, you may have insufficient immunity, so it should be adjusted and supplemented frequently. If your kidneys are deficient, your vitality will be insufficient, which will lead to deficiency throughout the body.

As you know, traditional Chinese medicine believes that the foods of the five colors nourish the five internal organs: red enters the heart, green enters the liver, yellow enters the spleen, white enters the lungs, and black enters the kidneys. Black beans have the functions of invigorating the kidneys, strengthening the body, and promoting blood circulation and diuresis. They are also detoxifying. Black beans are suitable for people with kidney deficiency. Regular consumption of black food not only regulates the physiological functions of the human body, but it also achieves moisturizing, beauty, and antiaging effects.

In winter, eat more melanin foods, such as black beans, black fungus, and black sesame seeds, which are good foods for strengthening the kidneys and strengthening the body.

However, people with acute nephritis and renal insufficiency, who have impaired ability to excrete metabolic wastes such as creatinine and urea nitrogen, should strictly limit their intake of low-protein foods and consume less of those grainy black foods.

You are as healthy as you allow yourself to be! Listen to your body and nourish yourself with the foods you need!

CHAPTER 6

Four Seasons of Health

"The best and most efficient pharmacy is within your own system."

– Robert C. Peale

According to the point of view that "human beings correspond to heaven and Earth," four qi refers to the four seasons of climate—spring, summer, autumn, and winter—that is: spring, warm; summer, heat; autumn, cool; and winter, cold. We should use reasonable means to adjust the spirit and emotions in order to achieve a healthy body and attain longevity.

The human body depends on the material conditions provided by the qi of heaven and Earth to survive. In spring, the liver should be nourished; in summer, the heart should be nourished; in autumn, the lung should be nourished; and in winter, the kidneys should be nourished. We should take good care of our spleen all the time.

Only by adapting to the changes of yin and yang in the four seasons, are the physiological activities of the five internal organs of the human body able to interact with the outside world. The world environment maintains a harmonious balance, which is basically consistent with the view of modern medicine. From the perspective of health preservation, these aspects are an inseparable whole.

In spring and summer, the climate changes from cool to warm, and yin declines and yang grows. You should do more outdoor activities so that the yang qi in your body can be more abundant. As you already know, there are three main activities that I recommend you do daily to achieve optimal health and wellness in all areas of your life: Tai Chi, yoga, and meditation. While I do not recommend meditating outside, Tai Chi and yoga are two great physical activities that you can do in your own backyard or even in the park.

In the autumn and winter seasons, the climate changes from warm to cool, and the yang disappears from the yin. We should pay more attention to preventing cold and keeping our body warm. Of course, there are the very obvious ways to keep warm, like keeping the temperature of your home regulated and wearing warm clothing, but there is also one way that people often do not think of.

In the Western world, so many people I have met drink ice water. While it may seem more refreshing, it is not good for your health. The best way to drink water is at room temperature, especially in the winter when you are trying to keep your body warm. But also in the summer, it is better for you to not drink cold water. Think about it this way: When you put cold water in a hot pot, what happens? It produces steam. Your body responds similarly. It is as if your cells are being attacked by the cold water. Start drinking your water at room temperature and you will see an improvement in your health.

Let me share a quick story about a friend, to show you what I mean:

Leilani has been a member of our meditation group for a very long time, and for as long as I can remember, she has struggled with her weight.

"You know, Celia, I try to eat better, healthier foods. I try to eat less, but it's just so hard. It seems like no matter what I do, nothing ever works."

"Do you want my advice, or do you just want to vent? It's okay if you just want to talk about it, without hearing what I have noticed. I don't want to offend you or make you feel bad."

"I know. It's just so frustrating. Everyone always has advice for me, but they don't know me."

"Yes, I know it can be annoying and that is why I asked."

In that moment, I was prepared to just let her share her frustrations with me, even though both my husband and I knew how she could help herself and that it was very simple.

"*Okay, Celia, I trust you. What do you think?*"

"*Well, I have noticed that often when we go out to eat, you choose a lot of deep-fried foods, and then after you eat, you wash it down with ice-cold water. This is very bad for your body. It is so unhealthy. If you can do one thing for yourself to start, it would be to drink your water at room temperature.*"

"*Wow. That is not what I thought you were going to say at all. I thought you were going to tell me to stop eating the deep-fried food.*"

"*Yes, you could cut down on that. Maybe if you let yourself have it once in a while, it would not feel like you are depriving yourself all of the time.*"

The next few times we went out for a meal together, I noticed that Leilani had not changed her habits, and a few months later, she developed stomach cancer. I know it can be hard to give up the foods that taste good and make you feel better, but it is all about developing new, healthy habits. You have to be ready to commit to the change. If you do not commit, you will not make it through the tough times.

On the days when you are struggling with eating better, lean on your meditations for help. The skills you are developing there will help you get through and stick to your health goals.

One last thing to think about when wanting to keep your body warm at any time of the year, is that public buildings often do not have their heat on high enough, or they are blasting their air conditioning. Always bring some layers with you when you go out, so that you can regulate your own body's temperature.

Eating and Drinking

It is of great significance to allow the nourishment of true qi, and to regulate the internal organs. Being too full or too hungry will damage the spleen and stomach to a varying degree, resulting in qi and blood disorders, causing related disease. People should have sufficient nutrition, eat and drink in moderation, and pay attention to the moderate temperature and coldness of their diets. The temperature of the food cannot be too hot or too cold, and the food should also be matched properly so that the spleen and stomach can be property nourished.

Always remember:
- In the spring, you need to nourish your liver.
- In the summer, you need to nourish your heart.
- In the autumn, you need to nourish your lung.
- In the winter, you need to nourish your kidneys.

Here are four more recipes to help you achieve optimal health in spring, summer, autumn, and winter:

Spring

Porridge

Ingredients:

Wolfberry 10 grams
Chrysanthemum 10 grams
olfiporia 20 grams
rice 1 cup
Salt 1 tsp

Instructions:

Clean wolfberry, chrysanthemum, wolfiporia, and rice.
Boil 6 cups of water, add all the ingredients to the boiling water, and cook for 30 minutes on medium heat.
Add salt according to your taste.

Benefits:

This porridge benefits the liver and kidneys. It also improves eyesight, has anti-aging properties, and helps lower blood sugar levels as well as blood pressure.

Summer

Stewed Duck with Winter Melon

Ingredients:

Winter melon 1000 grams
Duck meat 500 grams

Gorgon 30 grams
Semen coicis 30 grams
Oil 1 tsp.
Ginger slices 10 grams
Green onion 10 grams
Salt 1½ tsp.
white pepper ½ tsp.

Instructions:

Cut the duck into pieces, blanch the duck pieces, clean, and set aside. Cut the winter melon into pieces, remove the seed, and set aside. Heat up oil in a pan. Put ginger slices, green onion, gorgon, semen coicis, and duck into the pan, and stir fry until the duck is 80% cooked. Add 2 cups of water and winter melon and cook for 20 minutes until duck meat is cooked. Add salt and white pepper and cook for another minute.

Benefits:

This recipe helps the functions of the spleen and qi. It is a summer tonic delicacy.

Autumn

Gorgon Peanut Soup

Ingredients:

Gorgon 60 grams
Red dates 10 pieces
Peanuts 30 grams
Sugar 20 grams
Water 5 cups

Instructions:

Clean gorgon, red dates, and peanuts.

Boil water, and add gorgon, red dates, and peanuts into boiling water. After it is boiling again, turn to medium heat and cook for 30 minutes.

Add sugar after it is cooked.

Benefits:

This soup is great for the qi. It is especially suitable for the turn of summer and autumn when the spleen and the stomach is still weak. Eating this soup can strengthen the spleen and stomach, and increase body fluid.

Winter

Radish and Mutton Soup

Ingredients:

Radish 500 grams
Mutton 500 grams
Ginger 10 grams
Green onion 20 grams
White pepper 3 grams
Salt 2 grams (add more salt according to your taste)
Water 1.5 liters
Oil 1½ tsp.

Instructions:

Cut and clean radish; set it aside. Blanch mutton and cut into pieces. Heat up oil in a pot, and add ginger, green onion, radish, and mutton. Stir fry 5 minutes. Add water; use medium heat and cook 30 minutes. Add salt and white pepper; cook for another minute.

Benefits:

This soup can warm up the body, nourishing qi and blood. The radish has the effect of regulating qi, guiding stagnation, and clearing internal heat.

Daily Life

"Every morning's dew is a fresh breath of a new beginning."

– Jessica Edouard

People should have regularity in their daily lives, which can especially reflect in terms of work, rest, and clothing. When you achieve this, the yang qi in your body is in harmony with the yang qi in nature. This is the core value of every human being on Earth. If you have enough qi, your blood flow will be good, which provides energy and strength to the entirety of your body.

If you want to live longer, you must follow the movement of nature; the yang qi of the world moves with the rhythm of ebb and flow. When the sun rises, you should get up and start doing what you need to with your day. When the yang qi gradually declines as the sun sets, you should rest. Only by living a regular life can people contribute to good health and reduce the occurrence of diseases.

Again, you may find it difficult to adjust your habits at first, but keep working at it and you will feel a shift in your body and in your life. As you know, the three pillars I talk about multiple times throughout this book will help you:

The three ways of exercising your body and mind: meditation, yoga, and Tai Chi.

Get a good night's sleep!

Eat for your health.

When it comes to the first one, I know many people struggle to maintain a daily exercise routine. I often hear that people are too busy. Work and chores get in the way and take priority. I know this is easy to let happen. We have all been there. But when you make exercise a priority, you will always find a way.

Outside of meditating or doing yoga or Tai chi, there are other ways that you can maintain a healthy lifestyle, and they do not require that you carve out a section of time every day. These ways simply require that you make healthier choices. For example, have you ever stopped to look at the parking lot just outside of grocery stores and shopping malls? They are packed just around the entrances, while the back of the lot always remains empty. Why do you think this is? Because people make a choice to walk the shortest distance. Imagine if you chose to park in a spot that was furthest from the door every single time you had to run an errand? Sure, it will take a bit longer, but you will be building exercise into your daily routine, rather than compartmentalizing everything. As you begin to do this, it will become second nature to make choices that incorporate more movement into your daily activities.

Another great one is making the choice to take the stairs. Walk up rather than ride up the escalator or elevator. When you are at home, if you have to go downstairs to get something, walk up and down the stairs a couple of times before you bring the item back up with you.

You can also use this idea with meditation. You can take moments when you are forced to sit for a while—for example, while taking the bus or waiting for a friend to meet you—to stop using your brain for a moment. I do this regularly, especially when I fly from New York to Hawaii. For the entire nine-hour flight, I meditate. I am small enough to be able to cross my legs in the seat, but I know most people can't do this. This doesn't mean you can't do it. Close your eyes and focus in on your breath. Use the steps that I shared with you at the start of the book.

Meditation breathing:

- *Exhale to begin to get out all of the chi.*
- *Inhale deeply, pushing your chi down into your dantian. (Remember the feeling of your hands just below your navel.)*
- *When you inhale, hold your chi for 3 to 5 seconds.*
- *Exhale.*
- *Repeat this, 3 to 4 times.*

In your daily life activities throughout the year, you want to keep in mind what season you are in. This will help you understand how to better flow with the movement of the Earth. Eat to nourish your body, and sleep with the setting of the sun.

Do Not Work Rashly

My teachings are all about releasing your thoughts and allowing your mind to get quiet. STOP USING YOUR MIND! When your thoughts control all of your waking hours, it can cause you to become delusional. When you are delusional, you have an inability to distinguish between what is real and what is not real.

Delusion means chaos. Any work that goes against the rules and exceeds the limit can be called delusional, meaning that you might place unrealistic expectations on yourself for what needs to be done or what you can accomplish in a day. Labor is labor, including physical labor, mental labor, and housing labor.

Don't work rashly. People should work and rest in a reasonable manner, so as not to hurt their qi. Excessive physical exertion can easily damage the muscles and bones, consume the essence and blood, and affect your organs, which can lead to all kinds of sickness.

Illness is always caused by overwork, which is also a common phenomenon in today's society. Prolonged usage of your eyes hurts your qi, prolonged sitting hurts your flesh, prolonged standing hurts your bones, and prolonged walking hurts the tendons. So, you have to follow the principle of working tirelessly. Yes, working tirelessly! Meaning you have to listen to your body.

How do you listen to your body? The answer is easy: STOP USING YOUR MIND! Quiet the chatter and just listen. Practice listening daily. When you feel a nudge from your body, stop, listen, and take it seriously. For example, the muscles in your calves may feel oddly sore one day. This is your body telling you something. What is it telling you? Are you doing too much of something?

When you exercise, do not exercise just to say you did. Ask your body what it needs, and it will tell you. A lot of people think that they have to do everything fast. In a world that values productivity with greater financial reward, how can you remind yourself to slow down? Take time to move more softly and more lightly. Again, allow your body the gift of time to flow with the motion of the day.

If you find you did not sleep well in the night, remember to nap between 11 a.m. and 1p.m. if you nap for fifteen minutes during this time, it will be like having had napped for two hours. Make sure you rest well. Again, do not go through the motion of resting without intentionally allowing your body the rest it truly needs.

Do things that you love, to help you relax. Some of the things I do for myself in the day are:

I love calligraphy. It allows me to be creative in a soft, meditative way. I can feel my qi rejuvenating with each line I add to the page.

If you can't tell already, I absolutely love cooking! I intentionally bring myself into the moment of making a delicious dish by engaging all of my senses. The smells envelop me. The tastes make my heart happy. The feeling of creating something delicious makes my soul sing.

I love reading a good book. I give myself time in a place where I feel relaxed and comfortable. When my brain wants to rush to the next activity, I remind myself that I have set aside this time and there is nothing else I should be doing.

I also love singing. It gives me such satisfaction when I hit the right note, and there is always joy in the act of letting my voice create a beautiful sound.

A long walk in the mountains makes me feel more alive!

No matter what you do in the day, enjoy each moment. If you are working, enjoy your work. If you are exercising, enjoy the movement. If you are eating a meal, focus on the goodness that you are sharing with your body. Live with intention.

Adjust the Spirit

In today's fast-paced society, people often face a variety of emotions and feelings. Mood, worry, panic, and sadness are the human body's response to the external environment. It is an instinctive physiological response to a stimulus. As human beings, these vivid emotions, along with our desires, lead our daily actions.

If your reactions are too intense or persistent, it can cause yin and yang disorders, qi and blood disharmony, and organ dysfunction. For example, anger will hurt your yang qi. Try not to get too angry too often, because it will drain your energy and ultimately lead to poor health. As long as the yang qi can be maintained, we will have good health.

I know it is easy to tell you to not get angry. You might be thinking that it is in fact unhealthy to suppress your emotions. Do not confuse my telling you to not get angry, with suppression. What I am telling you to do is to deal with your emotions in a healthy way. When you feel triggered to anger by a situation or a thought, take a moment to breathe. Stop thinking; just focus on your breath. Remember, there is always a calm, rational, and intentional way to deal with anger. Give yourself time to release the chaos and to come to a place where you can think rationally.

When you experience a lot of anger, it can hurt your liver. Also, if your liver is unhealthy, it can lead you to anger. It is your liver that controls anger. If you feel that you have an unhealthy liver, try some of the recipes I have shared with you in this book, and also add more greens to your diet.

Sometimes when we feel we have lost our ability to communicate our feelings, this can lead to a buildup of anger and anxiety within the body. In this case, you want to open your throat chakra. Meditation and Tai Chi will both help with this. So will singing and making noise.

If you feel that you are quick to anger lately, or that you feel like you are living in a constant state of anger, try the exercise on the next page when you wake up in the morning.

- *Find a quiet place where you won't be interrupted, and you will feel comfortable making some noise.*
- *Sit ready to meditate.*
- *Close your eyes.*
- *Take a deep breath in. Push all of your qi to your dantian and hold for three seconds.*
- *When you exhale, make a shhhhhhhh sound, like you are telling someone to be quiet.*
- *Repeat the last three steps for five to ten minutes.*

To be in and maintain good health, you should reconcile your emotions. In doing so, you keep your mind at peace and quiet. Eliminate distracting thoughts; prevent violent fluctuations in emotions that interfere with the normal movement of qi. When you allow yourself to not get stuck in thoughts that steal away your energy, you create a good environment for gasification activities in the body.

The Flow of Life

Do you ever have those days when you feel like you are running on the spot? No matter what you do, you can't move forward. It is like you are one of those hamsters running on a wheel in a cage.

We have all had those days. I believe these happen when our desires, thoughts, or actions are out of alignment with the flow of our lives, our higher purpose. When you let your thoughts take control of every single aspect of your life, you do not leave space to listen—to listen to your body, to listen to your heart, and to listen to the world around you.

Trust that the universe, or God or a higher power, has your highest and best at heart. But if you are unable to listen, you won't hear the message. When I wake up in the morning I am flooded with ideas. I believe these to be messages from spirit. I stop and I listen. Is there anything I want to take note of? Is there any action I need to take today?

The mind controls the physical world; if it is too cluttered, there is no room for the messages from the spiritual world to break through, and you will experience poor health. The meaning of life is the combination of the spiritual and the physical. The spiritual world is the yin, and the physical world is the yang. Achieve peace by flowing with life, and ensure that your physical, emotional, and spiritual health is at its best in summer, fall, winter, and spring.

CHAPTER 7
The Difference Between Sleep and Meditation

"Our greatest human adventure is the evolution of consciousness. We are in this life to enlarge the soul, liberate the spirit, and light up the brain."

– Tom Robbins

Understand your brain and train it to work optimally in every situation you face in life. For most of us, this means knowing how to quiet it—how to stop using it in order to gain greater clarity, strength, and overall growth. It also means continuing to pursue knowledge even later in life. As you age, it is important to maintain balance in your daily activities, giving your mind time to focus, to learn, to think, to rest, and to heal.

I begin this chapter by sharing some basic information with you about the brain. You may know it already, and you may not. Either way, read it with the specific intention of understanding how to harness the power of both sleep and meditation in your life.

What Is Neuroplasticity?

"Neuroplasticity is the brain's capacity to continue growing and evolving in response to life experiences. Plasticity is the capacity to be shaped, molded, or altered; neuroplasticity, then, is the ability for the brain to adapt or change over time, by creating new neurons and building new networks.

"The importance of neuroplasticity can't be overstated: It means that it is possible to change dysfunctional patterns of thinking and behaving and to develop new mindsets, new memories, new skills, and new abilities."[2]

What does this mean? It's simple, really. If you want to keep learning, to keep growing, you need to do new things. For example, exercise is amazing for the brain. If you do not have an exercise routine, the best way to create one is to stay diligent. Set a time every single day to practice yoga or Tai Chi. The first time you practice, you will feel strange. Even simple movements will feel so foreign to your body. It may make you think, "I'm not good at this. I should stop." Or even, "This doesn't feel good. Maybe it's not right for me."

This is normal. Always listen to the messages your body is sending you, especially if a movement or a stretch feels like it is painful in a way that will cause injury or harm. That said, push through the awkwardness and the soreness you will experience in your muscles, to keep working at it. You'll notice, even after a few attempts, that the balance pose you thought would be impossible is easier than you thought. The repetition of this movement is establishing both muscle memory and a stronger pathway in your brain.

If you continue to work at your practice, you will find that you don't even have to think about it at all. You won't have to consciously figure out the movement or the pose. This is why both Tai Chi and yoga are so beneficial for not only your physical health but your mental health as well. They allow you those meditative moments that take you out of your active thoughts and, in a way, allow you to stop using your brain.

What Are Brainwaves?

Everything you do in your life requires some level of brain activity, even when you are sleeping; and yes, meditating. This is a good place to note that this book is called Stop Using Your Mind, not Stop Using Your Brain.

"At the root of all our thoughts, emotions, and behaviors is the communication between neurons within our brains. Brainwaves are produced by synchronized electrical pulses from masses of neurons

---

[2] https://www.psychologytoday.com/us/basics/neuroplasticity

communicating with each other.

"Our brainwaves change according to what we're doing and feeling. When slower brainwaves are dominant, we can feel tired, slow, sluggish, or dreamy. The higher frequencies are dominant when we feel wired, or hyper-alert."[3]

Types of brainwaves:

GAMMA

These are the fastest brain waves and are associated with learning new things, experiencing great insight or expanded consciousness, and moments of strong focus.

BETA

Beta waves are what we live in most of the time. They are not as fast as gamma waves. When your brain is operating in beta, you are productive and able to focus, which is where our current society, especially in North America, asks us to live most of the time.

ALPHA

Alpha brain waves hopefully jump in and allow you to relax at the end of the day. If you are unable to enter this slower state in your thoughts, you probably experience a lot of insomnia and anxiety.

THETA

You enter into theta when you sleep and meditate, although it can also be associated with peak performance when you are in a hypnotic flow state, like when you have mastered a Vinyasa series and can move through it without consciously thinking about your next step or the position of your body.

DELTA

When in delta, you are able to heal. This state completely removes the external world. You can be in this state both in meditation or when

---

[3] https://brainworksneurotherapy.com/what-are-brain-waves

you are dreamlessly sleeping.[4]

How Do Brainwaves Affect Your Health?

"Our brainwave profile and our daily experience of the world are inseparable. When our brainwaves are out of balance, there will be corresponding problems in our emotional or neuro-physical health. Research has identified brainwave patterns associated with all sorts of emotional and neurological conditions."[5]

Like I mentioned, when you are constantly over stimulated, it can lead to disrupted sleep and anxiety. Whereas, if you are operating at a lower brainwave consistently, it can lead to lethargy and depression.

How Can You Control Your Brainwaves?

I think the answer to this one should be an easy one to figure out at this point! Here are a few quick ideas to get you inspired:

- Create balance in your daily activities.
- Practice yoga or Tai Chi daily.
- Meditate.
- Learn new things.
- Make time to rest.
- Allow yourself to get a good night's sleep.

The Relationship Between Sleep and Meditation

"Wakefulness and sleep are like sunrise and darkness, while dreams are like the twilight in between. Meditation is like the flight to outer space, where there is no sunset, no sunrise—nothing!"

– Gurudev Sri Sri Ravi Shankar

Obviously, the brain is so much more complex than a thousand words can truly convey, but my hope is that the information I have

---

[4] https://naturesoundretreat.com/types-of-brain-waves/

[5] https://brainworksneurotherapy.com/what-are-brain-waves

shared here will help you understand how sleep and meditation are both related but different.

Both sleep and meditation provide your brain and body with the essential rest it needs for greater vitality and optimal health. You will never achieve your health goals if you do not rest. It really is that simple. When you regularly get a good night's sleep, you feel more energized, which inevitably allows you to be more productive, feel happier, and make healthier choices.

Similarly, meditation can lead to an improved mood, better memory, greater clarity of thought, and a stronger ability to focus. In Sanskrit, there is a term for the deepest level of meditation one can achieve: samadhi. In samadhi, your brain activity suspends completely.

"Samadhi is said to be a blissful and calm state of mind, in which the practitioner is no longer able to perceive the act of meditation or define any separate sense of self from it. In releasing the self from ego and the illusion of separation, samadhi is undisturbed by emotions such as desire and anger. As such, samadhi connects practitioners to their true self as one with universal consciousness."[6]

Scientific research has shown that samadhi and deep sleep are similar states in which the brain operates mostly in low frequency delta waves. So yes, deep sleep and meditation are very similar.

Some of the differences between deep sleep and deep meditation:
- A big difference is in the breathing. Once you reach samadhi, your breathing will become very slow and shallow. In deep sleep, while your breathing slows, it does not do so to the same degree.
- The main difference, and you may already have guessed it, is that when you meditate, you are actively remaining alert even though the alertness is very different from what you feel when you are simply going about your day.
- Meditation can be even more healing than deep sleep! Yes, you read that right. Meditating is so good for your body and brain, especially if you are able to reach that point when your brain stops doing all the work.

---

[6] https://www.yogapedia.com/definition/4995/samadhi

- The level of rest you achieve in meditation can be up to five times greater than deep sleep. This, of course, contributes to the last point.

Staying Awake in Meditation

Sometimes you may feel sleepy when you begin your meditation. This is completely normal. Do not beat yourself up or assume that meditation is not something you can do. Keep trying. Sometimes when one of our students feels sleepy, we instruct them to lie down for ten minutes and take a nap. After their nap, they often find they are more successful in their meditation.

If you are still having trouble, it is time to explore if the yin and the yang in your body are off balance.

"The yin is at rest while the yang is more active. Yin is growing while yang gives life. The yang transforms into the qi; the yin transforms into the material."[7]

You already know a lot of the ways you can help yourself achieve balance in both the yin and the yang. But here is a quick reminder.

In order to achieve the balance of yin and yang:

- I focus on my diet on a daily basis. I try to eat five different colors in my veggies and fruit. A balanced diet is essential for balancing the yin and yang energies within our bodies.
- When I eat, I do not let myself get to a point where I feel 100% full.
- I don't drink cold water and soda.
- I don't drink alcohol.
- I don't eat junk food at all.
- I go to bed at or before 10:30 p.m. If I have things to do at night, I would rather go to sleep early and get up early to do it in the morning. The good night's sleep relaxes my mind and replenishes my yin and yang energies. It also regulates my metabolism.

---

[7] https://zenitshiatsu.org/the-concept-of-yin-and-yang-and-the-body/

- I normally wake up at 5 a.m. to meditate, and I do yoga after meditation. I also go to the mountain in the morning, listen to the birds singing, and feel the fresh air. Another important thing is that I never spend even one second thinking about negative things. I will keep myself 100% positive. I won't let any outside environment violate my internal peace. I truly believe that the outside world is the reflection of my internal world.

Sometimes it is good to test if you are out of balance. One exercise that we often do with our class is to ask them to sit up straight and focus on their breath for five minutes. During this time, we observe if they are leaning to one side. If the body is leaning to the right or the left, it means that the qi on that side of the body is weaker. The qi needs to flow well throughout the entire body to be able to achieve a meditative state.

When this happens, we will redirect the class to move through the seven motions of yoga. If you are completing your own solo practice at home and are having a difficult time meditating because you want to fall asleep, try these seven motions and see if it helps you.

The Seven Motions of Yoga

The seven sections of lotus yoga were developed by Master Padmasambhava and provided by Master Wanxing. The goal of this series of movement is to elevate the natural qi of the human body, therefore giving it the opportunity to live in optimal health every day. The history of this series of movements goes back more than thirteen hundred years.

Section 1 – Guanyin Invites the Saints

This is a standing posture. Keep your feet as close together as you can without feeling wobbly.

Movement:

- Extend your hands, but make sure your arms are not too straight.
- Bend back while breathing in, and then reach your arms out to the

side while coming back to standing and exhaling.

- Imagine your hands are grabbing the edges of the universe on both sides at the same time.
- Place the palms together between the eyebrows (don't straighten them). Watch the universe merge into one energy ball.
- Squeeze your chin, straighten your hands up high, and lift the energy ball above your head. (The whole body is in a straight line perpendicular to the ground, and it is pulled straight.)
- Then open the palms slightly and pour the energy ball into the top of the head. (At the same time, imagine that your body is a bottle, and the energy fills up the bottle all at once.)
- Slowly open your palms from the top of your head and bring them down slowly in front of your face and then your chest, until they reach your dantian. Open your palms and exhale.

Note: The purpose of this exercise is to help your qi and blood flow smoothly. If done correctly, your hands should feel hot. Sometimes it can be difficult to understand a movement without seeing it. Here is a video of all seven movements to help you see what I mean. This video, performed by Master Wanxing, can be found at https://www.youtube.com/watch?v=mUXEy_qan6c

Section 2 – The Crane Spreads Its Wings

Stay in the same standing posture as you did for section 1.

Action:

- Use the energy in your shoulders to hold the arms.
- Use the energy in your arms to hold the hands.
- While lifting the arms out to the side, inhale, and lift the heels.
- Fill the breath and sink into the dantian.
- Focus your mind on the middle finger, which is the tip of the "wing."
- Hold your breath for 3 to 5 seconds, lower your arms slowly, exhale at the same time, and drop your heels.

Note: When you inhale, hold your breath in the dantian, and after the arms fall, exhale. The section helps the central meridian rise. It empowers the qi in your body while exercising the shoulders, elbows, and wrists. Your arms are like a crane spreading its wings, pulling the energy from the lower part of your body upwards.

Section 3 – River Stop and River Turn

This section also happens in a standing posture; but this time, spread your feet to be just wider than your shoulders.

Action:

- Raise both arms up so that your whole body is in an X shape.
- Bend backwards at the same time and inhale.
- After the inhalation is full, bend forward sharply.
- Take advantage of the trend to move the arms from between the feet, and throw them backwards, while exhaling.

Note: The power descends from your head to your toes, and the feet stand firm as if they were rooted. Breathe fully. From top to bottom, rely on the power of the waist to swing, and open the two veins of Renmai (conception vessel) and Dumai (governor vessel). This is a great exercise for curing back pain and can help to decrease abdominal fat accumulation. This section causes the fire of the heart to drop and the water of the kidneys to rise.

Section 4 – The Universe Rotates

Stay in the same standing posture as section 3.

Action:

- Cross your hands and five fingers.
- Make a circle with your arms. Lift your arms straight to the left, turn your waist, and inhale at the same time. From here, swing your arms to the top of your head and then press them down to the right.
- Bring the palms to the sides of the body and let the palms fall to the outside of the feet, on the ground, while exhaling.

Note: The rotation should always come from the waist and not the arms. Your arms will remain straight throughout. This exercise will soothe the liver and strengthen the kidneys. This action, along with the ones prior to this, helps to balance the yin and the yang, bringing balance to the power on the left and right sides of the body.

Section 5 – Rhino Watching the Moon

Stay in the same standing posture as section 3.

Action:

- Let both hands hang down naturally.
- Then raise the left hand upwards while inhaling. Imagine the force of the universe has been caught.
- Press down on the right and exhale at the same time, letting the tip of the left finger reach down to land on the inside of the right foot, the right hand naturally coming up. The eyes are guided by the right hand, up to the sky.
- Repeat this movement on the other side.

Note: You should never be too straight. Try to keep a bit of an arc shape to them. Your feet are like pillars of strength, so the knees should not be bent. This movement, combined with the earlier sections, will rotate and exercise your neck.

Section 6 – Lotus Swing

Go back to the same standing posture as sections 1 and 2. Remember to release your tension and let your arms hang down naturally.

Action:

- Rotate the lumbosacral region (your hips)15 times clockwise (to absorb energy), then 10 times counterclockwise (to release energy).
- Breathe naturally.
- Keep your shoulders as still as possible.

Note: At the beginning, the rotation range should be large so that the power inside will be activated. After a while, you can lessen the range of movement. This action replenishes the energy of the body.

Section 7 – Standing Up to the Sky

Stay in the same standing posture.

Action:

- Raise your shoulders, inhale at the same time, and lift your heels.
- Form your hands into hollow fists, like you are holding an apple in each hand.
- Keep your arms straight down.
- After holding your breath for three to five seconds, drop your heels (loudly), exhale at the same time, and release your hands.

Note: Keep your whole body vertical and your shoulders as high as possible. The circulation of your qi is from the back up and the front down, in a circular fashion. When you complete the movements of this section, you make the lotus flower (your head) open at once when the water (qi) flashes out from it.

Chapter 8

Healthier and Happier Every Day

"It's up to you today to start making healthy choices. Not choices that are just healthy for your body, but healthy for your mind."
– Steve Maraboli

In this book, I have shared with you the benefits of meditation for both your physical and mental health. I want to pull all of that together, along with a few more final points, so that you have it available to you in one easy-to-access chapter when you need it. Even if you have begun to develop your own practice while reading, and feel confident in it, there will be times when you face challenges. I hope this will be a helpful resource for you in these times.

I want to begin by reminding you of a very important lesson I shared all the way back in Chapter 2:

- Stress weakens your heart.
- Anger weakens your liver.
- Worry weakens your spleen.
- Grief weakens your lungs.
- Fear weakens your kidneys.

In order to feel healthier and happier in all areas of your life, it begins with the organs.

Meditate!

When you meditate, you achieve the goal of balancing these five organs. By meditating, you improve your chi and your blood flow, which in turn nurtures your internal organs, and the organs act like a nonstop factory to support and give balance to your life. With a strong heart, you can overcome stress. With strong kidneys, you can fight your fear. With a strong liver, you can take control of your anger and respond from a place of calm. But there are so many more benefits to finding balance within your organs. For example, if your liver is good, your body will be more flexible. When your liver is in a healthy condition, then the tendons will be soft.

Meditation has the power to give strength to your body to overcome the thoughts of the mind. One of the reasons we feel sick is because some organs begin to hold too much chi. When you focus on breathing into your dantian, sit in a good position, and give your mind a rest, you improve the flow of your chi and bring more balance.

Meditation Break

- Sit cross-legged, with either one leg on top or both legs on top of each other in a quiet, warm room. Set your alarm for 10 minutes.
- Exhale to begin to get out all of the chi.
- Inhale deeply, pushing your chi down into your dantian. (Remember the feeling of your hands just below your navel.)
- When you inhale, hold your chi for 3 to 5 seconds.
- Exhale.
- Repeat this, 3 to 4 times.

Allow your mind and body to sit in silence. If you find unwanted thoughts getting in the way, always come back to your breath. Always be kind to yourself. Your thoughts can be powerful and they do not want to be silenced. Try not to get frustrated with yourself. Just calmly come back to your breath.

Eat Nourishing Food!

A well balanced, healthy diet is at the core of well-being. Follow the theory of the five colors for your diet, and improve it by applying seasonal food. A balanced diet high in fruits and vegetables, lean protein, low-fat dairy, and whole grains is needed for optimal energy. Consume a variety of foods from all the food groups to get a range of nutrients.

Remember:

- **Liver** – Green food enhances the function of your liver.
- **Heart** – Red food enhances the function of your heart.
- **Spleen** – Yellow food enhances the function of your spleen (the digestive system).
- **Lung** – White food enhances the function of your lungs.
- **Kidney** – Black food enhances the function of your kidneys.

Get Enough Sleep

Remember to go to sleep at or before 11 p.m. If you don't get enough sleep during the night, try to take a rest and sleep for at least 15 minutes between 11 a.m. and 1 p.m.

Prioritizing sleep is one of the best things you can do to set yourself up for a healthier, happier, and energized day. Sleep deprivation can perpetuate serious health conditions and affect the balance of your chi. When the balance is off, it will affect your mood, motivation, and energy level.

I always hear my friends complain that they can't fall asleep right away after they go to bed. My suggestion is to observe your sleep patterns, and before you sleep, try to meditate for at least 15 minutes. Use the ways that I have mentioned in Chapter 4 to get a good sleep. With improved sleep quality, you will experience better health, feel happier, have improved emotional well-being, and lower your risk of disease.

Here is the brief summary of the 24-hour qi cycle:
- 3 a.m. to 5 a.m. is lung time
- 5 a.m. to 7 a.m. is large intestine time
- 7 a.m. to 9 a.m. is stomach time
- 9 a.m. to 11 a.m. is spleen time
- 11 a.m. to 1 p.m. is heart time
- 1 p.m. to 3 p.m. is small intestine time
- 3 p.m. to 5 p.m. is urinary bladder time
- 5 p.m. to 7 p.m. is kidney time
- 7 p.m. to 9 p.m. is pericardium time
- 9 p.m. to 11 p.m. is triple burner time (associated with the thyroid and adrenals)
- 11 p.m. to 1 a.m. is gall bladder time
- 1 a.m. to 3 a.m. is liver time

Practice Yoga & Tai Chi

Yoga is an ancient practice that combines mindfulness with physical movements to cultivate a balanced and healthy life. Practicing yoga on a daily basis can relax your mind, reduce stress, help you lose weight, increase flexibility, and improve balance. Overall, you will feel happier and sleep better!

Tai Chi has equally beneficial outcomes. Balancing the yin and yang in your body is an essential concept in Tai Chi. The pushing and pulling motions common to the postures are one example of utilizing yin and yang in this ancient practice. In Tai Chi, you emphasize precise biomechanical alignments and posture, helping your body move with more efficiency and less strain.

Tai Chi trains you to feel your body with increasing detail and depth. Once you develop greater awareness and sensitivity to your body, you begin to feel where you are holding tension, and then you begin to release the tension. Through practice, you pay more attention to the present moment, and you understand that each one is a unique moment in your life. It is one to be enjoyed without negative emotions from the past or anxiety for the future getting in the way.

Finally, both yoga and Tai Chi can act as a means of lowering blood pressure, increasing lung capacity, improving respiratory function, and boosting circulation and muscle tone.

Drink Water at Room Temperature

Seventy percent of your body is fluid. Drink room temperature water instead of ice water to keep the qi of your organs in balance. Water also flushes toxins and keeps your brain sharp.

Be a Lifelong Learner

Don't limit yourself from learning new things! Find something that interests you in life and keep learning. I am going to share with you some of the things I continue to learn about in my life, and I hope they inspire you to keep learning in your life. Learning not only gives you purpose but also a sense of accomplishment. It doesn't matter what age you are; learning keeps you young!

Here are some of my passions:

- Calligraphy
- Watercolor painting
- Oil painting
- Creating beautiful flower arrangements
- Tea ceremonies
- Cooking
- Singing
- Music

So, ask yourself: What do I love? What have I always wanted to learn about in my life but have held myself back? From here, take action! Find a course to get you started, or a group to join that will keep you inspired.

Learning is like exercise for your brain. "If you don't use it, you will lose it" applies here too!

Love Yourself!

*"Accept yourself, love yourself, and keep moving forward.
If you want to fly, you have to give up what weighs you down."*
-**Roy T. Bennett**

All too often, people tend to find love from another person. They need other people to love them. They care about how other people feel about them. Yet, I always tell my friends that love comes from within. When you love yourself, you are able to recognize your value and your own uniqueness. First learn to love yourself! When you love yourself, you will take good care of your spirit and your physical body. Then and only then will you be able to truly care for the ones you love.

I know that this is easier said than done. I could write an entire book on how to do the work you need to do to love yourself. But for now, recognize if this is work you need to do. Make a commitment to yourself to do it. Start finding resources. Read books, and research group coaching or individual coaching. Maybe a therapist might work better for you. Whatever you do, actively work on loving yourself every single day. You are important. Your life is important. LOVE YOURSELF TODAY!

Embrace Setbacks

No matter how much you prepare or how much you plan or how much you think you know, life will set you back. There is no way to avoid it. The thing that is most important is how you deal with setbacks. Do you bury your head in the sand and wait for it to go away? Do you whine about it? Do you let it take you down? Do you give up? Or do you face it head on? Do you allow each setback to help you grow stronger?

I told my son when he was very young that as a human being, you have to learn to accept setbacks and learn how to deal with them. Only when you know how to handle them, then you know how to endure life gracefully.

Plan for Success

Plan for success and take action on that plan now. When you know you will succeed, you are confident in your decision making. Rather than thinking about getting exercise, you will do it today. Rather than putting off eating better, you will be inspired to make different choices right away. Always remember that time waits for nobody. If you wait, it will be too late.

You are meant to thrive in your life. The universe is rooting for you to succeed. Today is the day! Change your mindset now and you will see results!

Take a Walk!

I love to walk in the morning. Sometimes I will meet a group of people at Diamond Head in Honolulu, and sometimes my husband and I hike up a mountain close to our home. My preferred time is between six and seven in the morning. It is such a beautiful way to start the day. I listen to the birds sing. I love being surrounded by the beautiful trees and plants. I always remind myself that living in the moment is the meaning of life. And I love these moments!

Find a place near your home that inspires you to get outside every morning to take a walk. If you can, invite a group of people to join. Many things in life are better with friends, especially when it comes to exercise. Having people join you will get you there on the mornings when it might feel easier to stay in bed!

Whatever you choose to do, get out there in the beauty of this world and have at least a forty-five minute walk every single morning. I promise that this one simple act will change your life!

Look at Life Through the Lens of Positivity

Always remind yourself that everything happens for a reason. When you can take each day and use what life throws your way as a lesson, you will begin to see things in a positive light.

Also, when you have a positive understanding of who you are, you will be able to face anything with strength, courage, and grace. No matter what happens, your positive attitude will guide you through, because you have allowed yourself to access the strength of your spiritual world.

Always remember that everything that exists or occurs in the physical world will end. Nothing lasts forever. The constant rule of this physical world is change. Therefore, you don't need to lament and regret what has already happened to you. Learn to embrace the bad and the good and enjoy this beautiful world. Breathe in the life-giving air. Look out at the beauty that surrounds you. Find gratitude for each moment of each day.

Get Creative!

One of the last pieces of advice I will share with you in this book is about creativity. As humans, we are called to create—create light, create joy, create delicious food, create products that make life easier, create stories that inspire, create life, create art!

You are a creative being. Allow that to shine through in your life. For me, I have found great joy in my paintings. It is a side of myself that I love sharing and am excited to share with you. I wanted to end this book in the most inspiring way I could think of, and I hope my art does that for you.

To see more of my work or to connect with me to see how we can work together, go to my website: https://www.celiakoart.com/.

Live Happy, Live Healthy!

www.ingramcontent.com/pod-product-compliance
Lightning Source LLC
Chambersburg PA
CBHW070537030426
42337CB00016B/2235